THE POWER OF POSTURE

Mindful Alignment for a Pain-Free Life

DR. RENU MAHTANI

Forewords by Hema Malini & Dr. K.H. Sancheti

JAICO PUBLISHING HOUSE

Ahmedabad Bangalore Bhopal Bhubaneswar Chennai
Delhi Hyderabad Kolkata Lucknow Mumbai

Published by Jaico Publishing House
A-2 Jash Chambers, 7-A Sir Phirozshah Mehta Road
Fort, Mumbai - 400 001
jaicopub@jaicobooks.com
www.jaicobooks.com

Editor: Meeta Kabra

THE POWER OF POSTURE
ISBN 978-81-8495-618-4

First Jaico Impression: 2015
Tenth Jaico Impression: 2018

Page design and layouts: Special Effects, Mumbai

Printed by
Snehesh Printers
320-A, Shah & Nahar Ind. Est. A-1
Lower Parel, Mumbai - 400 013

Dedication

*To all those who have taken charge of themselves
and have actively participated in their health and well-being.*

GRATITUDE

I thank the Divine for uniting me with yoga and for giving me innumerable opportunities to serve those in pain and help them discover the magic of awareness for living pain-free lives.

Doing the book was challenging and needed opinions and inputs of many that I could share, with utmost joy, every detail of yoga postures with lucidity. I am grateful and owe deep gratitude to each one of them.

I thank my loving family and dear friends who have encouraged and supported me in my quest to explore healing and health:

Dr Nagarathna from SVYASA, Bangalore, for guiding me to combine medical knowledge with the fundamentals of yoga. Dr Warren Reaves, FRCS Orthopaedics, the most revered osteopath and chiropractitioner, who is a role model of good posture. Your trust and blessings in this project have been invaluable; you have been an extraordinary mentor.

Surhuda Kulkarni and Devika Mundkur, for your expert inputs to my first draft. This project got the kickstart it needed because of your efforts.

Meeta Kabra, you were Godsend for the project. Being a content designer and yoga teacher, you understood the subject and put all your passion into enhancing it – a feat that you alone could have accomplished.

Anuradha Sule, for the monumental task of sketching my ideas into simple, comprehendible pictures. The readers will truly benefit from your illustrations.

My incredible team of yoga teachers – my second family; who

motivated me to bring out these simple yet effective concepts in the public arena. Many thanks to Dr Sanyogita Nimbalkar, Deepa Nair, Aakash Ramchandani and Anjeli Singh – our yoga teachers, for being the models in the photographs. Your poise, enthusiasm and smiling faces will be the biggest motivators for the readers. Vinay and Sanjay, for your remarkable talent through the lens and adding life to the photographs.

Last but the most important of them all, my clients, who have complete faith in me and without whose love and conviction, I would not have become a better person and a better doctor.

Thank you every one for making this project happen!

PROLOGUE

Living with awareness should be a way of life. Being aware of yourself helps feel well, look well and stay healthy. I learned this the hard way when a chronic and stubborn skin disease struck me. It prompted me to look for a holistic solution to a problem that was more than skin-deep. That is when the pill of awareness came into my life in the form of yoga. The varied physical practices and breathing exercises of yoga not only cured my skin problem, but also improved my general health and energy levels over time.

I also had a slight hunch on my back and suffered frequent neck and upper back pain. Sitting for long hours to study the voluminous medical text books added to the discomfort. I had been told that the hunch was genetic since my brother and uncles had it too. I took this to mean that I had to live with the hunch and accept that my aches would keep surfacing intermittently. Therefore, I never paid heed to the pain and continued racing with life with my distorted frame and associated aches.

The yoga practices prescribed for the skin disease started spilling out, off the yoga mat, into other aspects of my life. I carried the straight back posture to my office chair – keeping my head, neck and spine in one line. I also started sleeping correctly in tune with my physical axis, acknowledging Lord Krishna's words in the Bhagwad Gita –

Sama Kaya ShiroGreeva – Keep the head, the neck and the spine in one line.

Without any conscious effort, to my utmost surprise, the depth of my hunched back reduced. Needless to say, the nagging neck and upper back pain totally disappeared!

I then realized that being a doctor was my biggest strength and doing yoga my greatest passion. It was at this point in time that I decided to fuse the two so that I could share the age-old wonders of holistic living with all my very dear patients. I not only ventured out as a student to various yoga institutes for learning yoga in depth, but also started sharing its simple techniques with my patients as and when my medically logical and intuitive mind guided me.

I gained tremendous experience in treating a wide range of diseases from the simplest to the most critical ones and changed my treatment methods – from prescribing medicines to patients to getting them off prescriptions. I started bringing them to participate in achieving their own good health.

With my medical experience and formal training from four different yoga institutes in India and outside, I began yoga sessions for small groups based on their specific needs. In no time, these sessions for small groups took the form of an organization where different forms of yoga were offered according to the needs of the participating individuals.

The establishment of the organization meant an exposure to an even wider variety of health problems in patients ranging from 20 to 80 years. They came to the organization after being exhausted with the conventional prescriptions and hoping to receive holistic solutions. Yoga, a holistic science, is known to offer solutions for the most chronic diseases. It has not only given relief to my patients with chronic lifestyle diseases, but has also helped them look for solutions for their nagging physical pains. Many of my patients suffering from excruciating chronic pain were already doing physiotherapy or yoga, but their pains and aches persisted. To determine the cause of the pain, I would often ask them to perform their exercises before me. The demonstrations given by the patients became a turning point in my life as I began noticing that:

- People have different body frameworks, depending on gender, genetics, lifestyle and level of awareness.

- Patients who have experienced a particular type of pain in a specific part of the body cannot be prescribed the same set of exercises.

- People need to adapt themselves to exercises such that they meet the need of that particular body framework.

- People tend to overdo the exercises, both in the range of movement and in the speed. Overdoing a practice does more harm than good.

- Inaccurately performed physical exercises eventually do more harm than good, even to very physically fit and athletic individuals.

- Sedentary lifestyle destabilizes the baseline tone of our muscles; without regaining this tone, no pain will ever go.

Slowly, a mantra started emerging: How you do is as important as what you do.

In spite of having an exercise routine, the number of out-of-shape, round-shouldered white-collared professionals there are is shocking. Even people who are seemingly aware of their bodies do not actually have enough practical knowledge regarding how to carry themselves in commonplace activities.

The digital age has brought conveniences in our lives that are now necessities rather than luxuries. However, urbanization and industrialization coupled with mobile and other wireless devices have, in many ways, made us immobile. For the growing number of young professionals, work and life today revolves around computers, TVs, and mobiles. As a result, they end up with rounded shoulders, protruded heads, upper back humps, slumped gait and so on.

This lifestyle – intellectually challenging but physically sedentary and crippling – is responsible for back and neck pains, upper
back soreness, migraine, poor sleep and general irritability in
spite of technological advancements like ergonomic chairs. This
lifestyle has also created other major health risks including obesity
and flabby muscles that lead to a host of other diseases. That,
however, does not mean that we stop enjoying the materially-
driven world. It only indicates that we must teach ourselves to
enjoy it without hurting ourselves.

The ensuing chapters are an attempt to share my experiences
and learning with those looking for a comprehensive, healthy
living. So, flash 'OPEN SESAME' to the awareness that the
following pages bring and they will unravel a treasure trove of
health that you wish you had known long ago.

Dr Renu Mahtani

FOREWORD

I had the good fortune of reading *The Power of Posture* written by Dr Renu Mahtani. It gives me great pleasure to write a foreword for this unique and much-needed book.

The book contains sound and practical advice, and a message, not only for elderly people, but for teenagers and adults too – that core yoga for a perfect posture is the key to good health and a pain-free body lifelong.

A good posture is the outcome of balance of strength and flexibility in the muscle groups. Without these, no treatment modalities can show the desired results. I appreciate the effort Dr Mahtani has taken in sharing the minutest detail on yoga postures in this thought-provoking book.

Aches and pains are constant reminders that we need to stop taking our body for granted and take action because they occur irrespective of all ages and recur like a nightmare when neglected for too long. X-rays, MRIs, physical therapy, surgery and so on... the options are all too many, but why wait to reach this stage when all one needs to do is practise simple exercises!

Dr Renu Mahtani's mission statement as a practising physician and yoga therapy consultant speaks rightly about 'how you do' being more important than 'what you do.' Just as we have evolved and changed from a physically active to a sedentary and comfort-driven society, yoga therapy too has widened its branches and does not confine itself to merely the perfect headstand or a series of difficult postures.

Yoga is not a one-size-fits-all protocol for everyone. The need of the hour is a logical understanding and application of yoga with appropriate adaptations, depending on the individual – the approach to women's problems has to be different from men's as women and men differ in muscle tone and strength. Yoga therapy is not just about flexibility; rather it is flexibility on the foundation of strength. This means mindfully using the breaths and core muscles before stretching the peripheral ones.

The Power of Posture also has simple yoga and pilates exercises that can be safely recommended to not only alleviate pain but also improve the core tone and metabolism; it may surprise many that low metabolism can be tackled with core tone! Yoga is a daily life-server for the well-being of the body, mind and soul. All techniques of yoga, when applied mindfully and round the clock, can become a healthy practice that can ensure an energetic body, toned-up physique and a pain-free living.

I believe that Dr Renu Mahtani's dedicated efforts will continue to motivate people and spread awareness to enhance every individual's lifestyle.

Once again, I applaud Dr Renu Mahtani for the wonderful book she has authored.

Best wishes and good luck to her for all her future endeavours.

Padmashree, Padmabhushan,
Padmavibhushan Dr KH Sancheti

Chief Orthopaedic Surgeon
Sancheti Hospital and Centre for
Joint Replacement Surgery, Pune

FOREWORD

One of the most practical books on daily yoga – this was my thought after I read the content of this elaborate research work to be published as a book, and for which Dr Renu Mahtani approached me to write the foreword.

I have read numerous books on yoga, pranayama and their practice and benefits. However, Dr Renu Mahtani's book, *The Power of Posture*, is one of the most insightful reads on yoga – it is a complete know-how on how to live holistically through yoga, 24 hours a day.

Being a classical Bharatnatyam dancer myself, I have always held the right posture, as this has been an integral part of my classical dance training. I believe the techniques employed in dance and yoga are similar in more aspects than one – through exercises or mind-body work outs. This book has given me a great insight on how useful my posture has been till date in my daily routine and has also educated me on how to care for my entire body, as I believe that this body of ours, is the most precious GIFT of God.

Not only does this book highlight the benefits and maintenance of a perfect posture through various asanas, it also explains how to sleep right, manage weight, and recover from illnesses, and puts to rest the various myths attached to our health at every stage of life. Dr Mahtani stresses the importance of a proper gait and simplifies the application of yoga in every aspect of our daily lives.

Having gone through this extensive piece of work, written in a lucid language and accompanied by comprehensible illustrations,

I no longer practise yoga for a scheduled work-out time merely. Instead, I have started applying the techniques highlighted in this book in just about everything I do.

Our work culture and lifestyle today are of a very demanding nature. Young students as well as working professionals are constantly striving to cope with stress and its ill-effects. This book caters to the needs of young adults who Dr Renu motivates to be in the best of spirits and health by including yoga in their lives. In fact, I would say that this book is a must for the youth.

The Power of Posture is a commendable piece of research work by Dr Renu Mahtani and I wish her the very best for its publication.

Padmashree, Padmabhushan Hema Malini
Member of Parliament, Actor, Dancer, Filmmaker

CONTENTS

Section 1

BLUE PRINT

Mindfulness is the miracle by which we master
and restore ourselves.
~ Thich Nhat Hanh

Chapter 1

AWARENESS WITHIN

Crises and deadlocks, when they occur, have at least this advantage that they force us to think.
~ Jawaharlal Nehru

What do we commonly do in the face of pain and unease? We rightly decide to go to the family physician for an opinion, which more often than not leads us to the x-ray room. In such cases, the diagnosis is usually made based on radiological findings. Often, heavy medical terminology is used to describe what has gone wrong – early osteophytes, increased lordosis, mild to moderate degenerative changes and so on.

Who among us would not be aghast by these diagnoses, especially when a second, or even third, opinion confirms them? Deep down, we are petrified because, for most of us, degeneration is almost comparable to a taboo. Rightly so, because degeneration does mean premature aging. And who wants that?

The wake-up call has been sounded. What next? Anxiety follows, with baffling questions. Doubts and confusion bog us down: I am only in my early 30s. Can aging set in so early? What is this degeneration? Is it really a disease? Is it that bad? Could I have possibly prevented it? Is it possible to reverse it or halt its progression? What did I do wrong?

The good news is that degeneration is not a disease; it is a disorder and, in most cases, a curable one. Degeneration of the body begins with the improper use of joints that bear the body's weight. Let us understand a few things about how weight-bearing joints, like those of the legs and the back, work. We also need to understand how we unknowingly participate in their malfunctioning. Only then will we be able to help ourselves and keep the body happy and free of pain.

Natural Equilibrium of Joints

The human body is a geometric combination of right proportions. Each bone has a natural slot that allows the adjoining bone to fit neatly into it. All the bones work at their optimum level when they are correctly aligned with each other and slotted properly in their joints.

Bones are made of hard material. As such, they are not supposed to rub against each other in the joints. To prevent this rubbing, nature has given them softer protective cushioning in the form of cartilage, that prevents abrasion at the joints.

Every weight-bearing joint in the body is in a state of perfect equilibrium. Nature enables this balance by providing strong muscles to hold the bones in place. Each joint also receives strength from adjoining muscles to balance the stress we put it through. Equilibrium occurs when the bones, the joint and the muscles are in a certain alignment – that is, through the center of the said joint. This enables us to handle and enjoy our day-to-day activities with ease and prevents wear and tear to the joint structure.

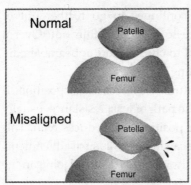

Joint between the thigh bone (femur) and the kneecap (patella)

Disturbance in the placement of the joint structure causes an imbalance. This happens when we do not use our muscles correctly, and they become too weak or too tight. Overuse, underuse or wrong use of muscles causes a shift in the weight-bearing axis of the joint, pushing it from the centre towards the side. This imbalance disturbs the cushioning between the bones, making the bones rub against each other and causing friction. If the imbalance becomes habitual for a person, it leads to constant gritting and rubbing of joints, which further leads to aches and pains, and in long-term cases, to functional aging or degeneration.

Pain: The Body's Signal

Our body gives us clear warning signs of such degeneration by triggering pain. However, most of us tend to ignore these early signs and symptoms. We continue with our daily physical activities, hoping that the pain will disappear on its own. When it does not, we take to pain killers and sooner or later become addicted to them, little realizing that they only suppress the body's cry for attention.

Taking Refuge in Comfort Zones

Slowly but steadily, the joint continues to go further out of alignment, causing the cartilage to reduce or thin out. Over a period of time, we are subjected to chronic and unbearable pain that eventually turns into disabling pain.

When in pain, the body naturally seeks a relief position. It finds a comfort zone by taking the path of least resistance, usually a tilt to one side, or some other position that reduces pain. This may be more damaging than one can imagine, as such adjustments tend to worsen the condition of the already damaged joints in the long term.

To compensate, the bones' edges at the joint begin to outgrow. They form tiny projections or spurs called osteophytes. These start to bear the weight of the body, which then stops passing through the centre of the joint. The spurs intrude on the joint space or on the nerve endings, where they do not belong, thus not only triggering more pain but also weakening the entire system at the point where the spurs occur.

Muscles Need Attention

We often ask ourselves: What is the point of counting the number in the flock when it has flown away? OR What is the point of repentance when the damage has been done?

Fortunately, this is not applicable to musculoskeletal disorders. Even when the damage is visible on an x-ray, the principles of healthy muscle use, posture alignment and focused exercises surely work! In over 25 years of my medical practice, I have seen innumerable patients with 'bad' x-ray reports living absolutely pain-free lives. More important and ironically, I have seen many more with normal x-rays who are suffering from severe discomfort and pain.

X-rays show only the imprint of the bones and the joints, but they cannot probe the muscle condition nor tell us about their functional status. Patients with bad x-ray reports are taught the basics of correct alignment. They apply these principles to maintain correct posture and are consequently able to maintain the health of their muscles and remain pain-free even with abnormal x-rays. Those who are not inclined to maintain their muscles' health continue to suffer with pain and disability in spite of normal or borderline x-rays.

In complex cases of joint problems, surgery is necessary. It is interesting to note that even highly advanced surgeries, like joint replacement, come with a prescription of dos and don'ts; most related to muscle work around the concerned joint. Any negligence in the recuperation period is likely to cause a relapse. Observations prove that an artificial joint may perpetuate the problem if the supporting muscles are not kept strong and supple.

Note that neither painkillers nor x-rays have solved the problem, nor has surgery freed anyone from taking care of themselves.

So, let's revisit the chain of events caused by some reason unknown to us. This is what it will look like in most cases:

Misaligned joints → Nagging pain → Painkillers →
Repetitive pain → X-rays →

Self-adjustment to a 'relief' position → Further misalignment → Osteophytes or some other compensation → Unbearable, disabling pain → Surgery → Most likely, lack of muscle care → Pain

Think before You Gulp

Doctors prescribe painkillers and anti-inflammatory medicines to relieve pain. While the medicines reduce inflammation and help mask the pain, they do not offer logical, long-lasting solutions to the problem. We continue popping pills, little realizing that by masking the pain, we are dealing with the problem merely at the superficial level and are only preventing investigation of the root cause.

Answers Lie Within

It's time to stop, think and ask: Can we do something, other than using chemicals, to stay pain-free? Is there a long-term solution around that we do not know of?

Habits compel us to seek complex, often harmful, solutions to simple problems. We have to admit that we are taking the easier route. After all, painkillers do allow us to continue with our perennially wrong habits. Some of us even opt for expensive surgeries! By doing so, we assume that we do not need to change ourselves. Of course, there are times when medicines may be a necessary evil. But we owe it to ourselves to look for deeper causes for our physical ailments and look for holistic approaches to resolve them.

We have to understand that taking painkillers as a habit leads to a partial loss of oneself; they create a disconnect between the mind and the body. If pain is suppressed, it does not allow you to assess the depth of the underlying problem. This casual attitude needs to be altered by showing respect to the great physical form; our body.

It is very likely that no one guided us so far. If the experts advising us believe that painkillers are the only solution, we cannot blame ourselves all the way either. What is required, then, is a patient and careful reassessment of our habits.

Pill of "Awareness"

Healthy muscles and healthy joints are like two souls living and working in tandem and harmony, wherein both need love, care and nurture. Merely replacing an aching joint does not suffice. Modern medicine is still not competent to manufacture artificial muscles or pills capable of synchronizing the working of the muscles with the nervous system. Even if you choose to go under the knife, there is no end to how much you can grow with more awareness. If you do not pay adequate attention to yourself, you are going to end up with the same problems, all over again.

Our present day healthcare system is elaborate and refined, and yet plagued by many 'buts' and limitations. It cannot replace 'awareness' – a vital source of our well-being – that we need to possess about our health. There is unfortunately no pharmaceutical pill to generate awareness.

What is 'Awareness'?

We begin with understanding how the body is naturally meant to be. We teach ourselves to look at ourselves physically, as someone else who loves us and cares for us. We assess our habits that are responsible for our present problems or have the potential to create issues in the future. When we have awareness at this level, it is half the battle won. A look at our physical selves impartially will create within us an interest for ourselves. We will then get absorbed in the deeper sense of being.

We are now ready to learn and address the true underlying reason – our posture. We will then retrace our way back to good body dynamics and solve present and future problems.

Chapter 2

WHY DO WE NEED A GOOD POSTURE?

A good stance and posture reflect a proper state of mind.
~ Morihei Ueshiba

As a teenager, while being engrossed in studying, I would end up slouching in the chair and my mother would repeatedly ask me to straighten up. The admonition made me correct my posture by over-lifting my chest, which in turn overarched my lower back and jammed my shoulders. Since I was unable to sustain this 'un'natural position, I would go back to slouching. My mother meant well, but only straightening up was not enough.

Good posture is not only about straightening up, but also about how we sustain our body in different positions and movements. It is about well-synchronized body parts that create graceful, flowing movements with minimum effort and maximum efficiency. Good posture allows our body to function optimally at all levels and does wonders to our energy and confidence.

Research corroborates that physical pain is caused by genetics, inadequate physical fitness, age, being overweight, smoking, osteoporosis and arthritis. However, years of medical practice have led me to trace the root cause of most pains to *bad posture* – faulty body dynamics in routine activities and also while exercising.

Patients, with physical aches and pains arising from poor posture, have experienced relief with postural corrections prescribed for their body types. Postural corrections have also led to toned muscles and a slimming effect, thereby rendering a confident and radiant demeanour.

It is imperative for the present and the future generations to focus on correct posture and body alignment to avoid succumbing to more musculoskeletal change. To wise up to the benefits of a good posture is the key to a graceful and healthy living and is the answer to curing most aches and pains. A few simple yoga techniques and lifestyle changes can make the journey of life a pleasant one.

It is vital to listen to our inner voice – the captain and life guard of our existence – in order to reap the fruits of a cheerful and warm presence, poise and a confident walk. Maintaining a correct posture goes a long way in keeping our lives pain free; physically, emotionally and mentally – and lends a slimming effect to our carriage, boosting our morale.

Appearances Speak Volumes

When we meet someone for the first time, subconsciously, posture is the first thing we notice about them. We judge them by their posture and the first impressions that we form of them tend, to become the lasting ones. People who slouch and slump look tired, clumsy, shorter and diffident, and are thought of as having an inferiority complex. In sharp contrast, those who have a good posture look taller, leaner and more alert, and are perceived as confident people.

Exude Confidence

People with a good posture radiate confidence, health and vitality, whereas a slouch projects insecurity and weakness. Improving the posture helps build self-esteem and improves our performance. Good posture conveys the message: I respect myself and helps command respect from others.

Boost Metabolism

A good posture not only makes you look attractive but is also scientifically proven to boost metabolism. To maintain a correct and good posture, we need to use the spinal and the core muscles with a little more tone than their baseline tone. This additional push to the muscle tone activates the idling metabolic pumps and helps burn the excess fat. Our postural muscles effectively work on the slump and slouch.

Take Inches off Your Waist

Simply standing straight can instantly slim the waistline by one to two inches. Try it out! Place a measuring tape around your waist as you sit with a slouch. Now, sit up straight and take the measurement again. You will be surprised.

Add Inches to Your Height

Forward slumping can decrease the height by as much as two inches. The good news is that one can regain the lost height by correcting the posture with the Instant Alignment Technique. (Refer to page 169, Chapter 18.)

A good posture is not just about standing erect or sitting tall but also about the position from which movements begin and end. It comprises the finer nuances of what we are doing or not doing with our body at a given time. The body is designed to work at its optimum level by maintaining a proper postural coordination between different body parts. This enables the body

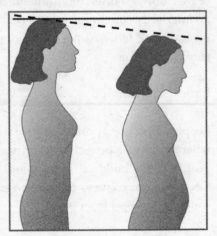

Height and posture

to perform movements with grace, thus reducing the strain on the joints and muscles.

Maintain Joint Health

Correct posture extends beyond an enviable figure; it is a dynamic force. With the correct posture, the bones and joints need not do all the hard work, as the muscles working evenly counter the gravitational force that pulls our body and bones down. When the deep stabilizing postural muscles work to maintain tone and support to the joints, the muscles for movement can work with maximum efficiency and strength to help the joints move with lightness. Through good posture, the proper use of muscles continuously supports the skeleton effectively and reduces the chance of injury and pain.

Improve Breaths

There isn't a better way to understand the immediate impact of posture than its effects on the breath. Try the following exercise to see how posture affects breathing pattern:

• Close your eyes, sit with a slump and observe your breaths.
• After a few breaths, sit up straight and observe your breaths.

Did you notice a change? The breaths are deeper and longer with a straight posture. This happens because the rib cage has expanded to create more space to accommodate air replete with oxygen. Improved quality and quantity of every breath directly translates into good health. Through improved breathing, correct posture adds vitality to the renewable life force that sustains us and helps reduce stress.

Keep the Heart Happy

Good posture opens up the constriction of the rib cage. This expansion facilitates improved breathing by increasing oxygen supply to the heart muscles, and the result is a stronger, healthier heart. Not only do good posture and right breathing help with chronic heart problems and prolong our life-span, they also make life fuller as the 'feel good' factor percolates to every cell of the body.

Digest Efficiently

Neurological-muscular disharmony causes medical conditions such as irritable bowel syndrome, constipation and bloating. Good posture improves circulation to the internal organs while stimulating the coordination of the nervous system. A proper posture decompresses the intestines, improving digestion. All abdominal organs function better as they have room to breathe.

Exercise Effectively

Workouts with an engaged tone and posture alignments yield best results. They make the motions of exercise comfortable and safe. On the one hand, you can exercise for longer durations with less fatigue, on the other, the resilience of the muscles and the joints improves, making them prone to fewer injuries. A good posture enables better breathing and increased oxygen intake. This is especially important for an intense exercise routine where the body gasps for oxygen, the deprivation of which can cause dizziness in the short run and more serious harm in the long run.

Develop an Alert Mind

Muscles cannot work without proper signals from the brain and the nerves. As we train our muscles to work well, dormant areas of the brain are activated, enhancing creativity and functional productivity. It is rightly said: Concentrate on keeping the spine upright to keep the brain alert.

Build Mental Strength

A proper posture necessitates an engaged mind. It involves connecting with our spinal and mental cores. Be it standing with the navel in or walking consciously with toned hip muscles, all these actions are mediated through the nervous system and the brain. Being connected through our body and breaths helps us look bright, stabilizes mood swings and offers comfort and solace during difficult times. The result is clarity of thoughts and emotional stability.

Get an Even Skin Tone

Right posture, in any activity, tones muscles and burns the fat below the skin. When the body is in the correct posture, the skin is uniformly stretched and all areas receive an equal amount of blood supply thereby rendering the skin supple and wrinkle-free.

Look Younger

Older people with good posture are perceived to look younger than their age. A study conducted in the United States showed how posture alters the perception of age. Two women of the same height but different body weights were asked to cover their faces. Side profile pictures of both were taken – one picture with a slump and another with a normal posture. The two appearances were then rated by 60 people. When they stood straight, they were consistently rated as younger and more attractive. The upright heavier woman was rated younger than the slumping thinner lady.

Live Life Pain-Free

Good posture can prevent a lifetime of annoying and painful problems at the weight-bearing joints of the body. With poor posture, the joints are misaligned, causing abrasion and pain even while performing simple day-to-day activities. Applying the basics of good posture helps balance the supporting muscles around the joints and the body moves with ease and comfort.

Maintaining a good posture may seem like a herculean task, but is in fact very simple, for:

A perfect posture is not one of being at military attention; it is one of keeping the body in a natural, relaxed alignment.

Chapter 3

OUR STORY – COMMON POSTURAL HABITS

We are all sculptors and painters. Our material is our own flesh, blood and bones.
~ Henry David Thoreau

Vinay is a young man in his thirties. When in college, he became an avid reader and was fascinated by computers. As his career flourished, he considered physical activities a waste of time. By the age of 35, he was a successful engineer but was also a victim of shoulder and neck pain. The pain was often so disabling that he had to take time off from work. His confidence dropped as he worried about aging.

Sounds familiar? Don't we or someone we know have similar complaints?

Ronak, Vinay's cousin, considers Vinay his mentor. At 25, he is as smart and successful as Vinay. It hurt him to see Vinay in such pain. Younger and wiser, Ronak wanted to find a way to relieve Vinay of his pain and to make sure that he wasn't himself susceptible to similar pains. Several doctors were consulted and x-rays done until a solution was found. It amazed Ronak to see how simple the solution was.

All Vinay needed to do was correct his posture and all Ronak had to do was adopt the same postural habits to prevent the pain. Knowing he is in control, Vinay now has renewed confidence. Even if the pain resurfaces, he knows what to do. Ronak has made preventive action a part of his daily routine and hasn't had to experience Vinay's pain personally.

In most cases, the root of aches lies in our habits. We tend to pick up damaging habits unconsciously and only later realize the damage caused. Since these habits are unconsciously adopted, it is not easy for us to correct them.

It is common knowledge that old habits die hard and that we are slaves to them. But there is hope. Habits become easier to mend when we know their root cause. Postural habits can be easily rectified if we are aware of them. Once identified, we need to be proactive about correcting those habits. Even a slight correction in posture leads to a more self-assured gait and a glowing personality.

We need to pinpoint the exact postural habits that may be the source of our pain or that are draining our energy. Let's start by understanding how our quotidian activities – walking, sitting, sleeping and bending forward – can cause physical imbalance and result in pain. I request you to not be afraid of the list of aches described in the successive chapters. This comprehensive list of pains is accompanied by an equally inclusive list of possible solutions.

Standing Habits

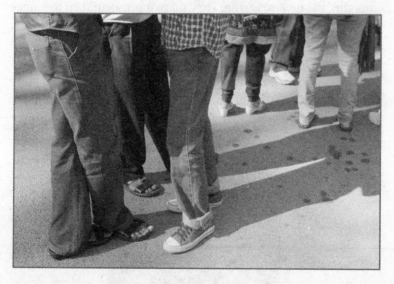

Some faulty standing postures

As humans, we are blessed with a strong central structure that enables us to stand and function on two legs, unlike creatures in the animal kingdom. Our feet act as balancing pads, which leave an impression on rubber footwear with constant use. These impressions reveal the pattern of uneven weight distribution on our feet. An ideal weight distribution is one where the weight of the body is evenly distributed on the right and the left feet, as well as the front and the back of our legs. For each foot, the weight should be borne equally by both the inner and the outer edges of the foot.

Standing for a long period of time is a painful activity for many of us, often causing severe pain that hurts the back, the knees and the feet. There are various reasons for such discomfort.

Uneven Weight on the Feet

For most people, the general tendency is to put more weight on the outer edge of the feet as compared to the inner side. For people with flat feet and knock knees (knees pointed inward rather than straight), the reverse is true. They place more weight on the inner edges of their feet.

We are also inclined to put excessive pressure on our heels by distributing the weight to both heels and the mounds of our soles (we are generally less aware of the mounds of our soles, the parts of the soles that would be on the floor if we were to stand on our toes). We rarely ever put any weight on these mounds and they stay mostly unused.

The Wide V Standing Posture

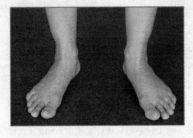

Wide V standing posture

The picture above shows a common standing posture where in we stand with the feet wide apart, wider than the span of the hips. In this posture, we also rotate our feet outward, which increases the distance between the toes of the two feet and results in locked knees. The locked knees are forced backward to cause immense strain on the knees and the supporting muscles.

The uneven distribution of weight on our feet and the V posture trigger a chain of reactions at the joints in our legs – the ankles, the knees and the hips. With time, the heels and the other parts of the feet that take the pressure, affect these joints negatively to damage the natural protective cushions around our bones.

The Best Foot Forward

We begin our walk with the same foot every time – left or right. We cannot be blamed for putting our best foot forward, but this habit can become a source of imbalance. If the best foot is the right one, it usually stays forward and the left foot is used to stabilize the body. This restricts the forward foot's movement. Even when we stand casually, the rear leg is the weight bearer. Even distribution of weight between both feet is a must.

Belly Hanging Out

The tight jeans that slim women wear camouflage the soft, flaccid and under-toned belly, causing the stomach muscles to slacken, which leads to displacement of the abdominal organs and the lower back over a period of time. This also results in unnecessary strain on the lower back. Such women need to build or tone their abdominal muscles. If corrective action is not taken, they may eventually end up with a thickened waist, a protruded belly, an over-arched lower back,

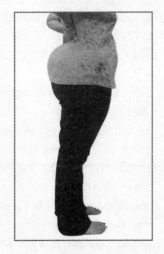

Weak belly, strained back

hunched shoulders, and complaints of back pain, soreness in the shoulders, and digestive as well as urinary problems.

Walking Habits

Walking, an extremely useful activity with loads of benefits, is also a rejuvenating aerobic exercise. A brisk walk makes for a good cardiovascular exercise along with toning and stretching the muscles of the lower body. While proper footwear is mandatory for walking, the most important thing to bear in mind is a good posture involving the core muscles of the body. Discussed below are some common faulty walking habits that we tend to see among people.

Dragging Gait

A drag in the walk is a common phenomenon due to poor muscle tone. The inability of the muscles to lift the limbs properly makes them seem heavier and creates an abnormal movement of the legs. The drag is more pronounced on the rear leg. The hips loosely sway from side to side due to toneless buttocks. Due to a toneless back, the chin bobs ahead, leading to a rounded back and shoulders. Overall, it appears that the body is burdened down.

Flip–Flop Gait

Ah the flip-flop! We instantly picture the cool and casual look of the flip-flop slippers – the vogue these days among the young crowd. Our feet are at ease in these V-shaped slippers. However, constantly wearing them aches our feet. The slippers though are not at fault; it is the V standing and walking that causes the aches and pains. While walking, the waddle of the feet also renders a V-shaped walk. This kind of walking places more weight on the heels and the outer edges of the feet and results in our knees getting locked and the joints getting pressurized. The constant locking of the knees forces our belly forward so that we end up with an exaggerated curve of the lower back. All that the V-shaped walking does is cause knee and back problems for the youngsters.

Over-Emphatic Heel Strike

Some people walk with an obvious thud in their walk due to a strong heel strike. The thud on the treadmill is even more pronounced. When we walk, most of us land on our heels, which puts undue weight on the knees. To counterbalance the pressure on the heels, we can adjust our walking by having a strong push off from the toes. This not only protects the knees, but also makes the step light and the walk buoyant.

Using the pushing-off-with-the toes technique while walking is beneficial for the spine. Unfortunately, this walking technique is underutilized.

Sitting Habits

Squatting on the floor to sit, a norm earlier, is now a redundant practice in India. We are now a civilization of chair users. As late as the last century, men would sit cross-legged on a cotton-filled cushion called *gaddi*, to conduct business, while women would sit on a slightly raised stool called *takhti*, to cook. People sat on the floor to eat meals. Today, sitting on the floor is an impossible feat for many Indians. Sitting on a chair has changed the entire relationship between our muscles and bones.

Ergonomic furniture, a new concept in the research and design of furniture to match our body types, is a new corporate fad. This furniture is programmed to offer the highest level of comfort. Unfortunately, it has robbed our muscles of their strength, leading to many postural problems with long-term damaging effects.

Sitting with Crossed Thighs

One thigh crossed over the other while sitting on a chair is an iconic pose. Remember Marilyn Monroe – she looked her glamorous best in this pose.

When sitting in this pose, as a habit, we cross our best leg over the other one. The upper leg twists in an outward direction, putting undue strain on the already lax knee structure. In women, the crossed thigh pose impacts the knee of the best leg with pain due to the flaccid and weak knee muscles. In men, with tight knee muscles, the impact is on the knee of the lower leg, as it bears extra strain and weight of the leg placed above.

Rounded Back

We have all observed pictures of ancient Hindu hermits at peace in the 'straight back' posture – the meditative pose. Their bodies are in an L shape, with the legs crossed on the floor. The ancient man never sat on chairs, especially in the Asian and African cultures. Research has shown lower rates of spinal damage in societies that squat or sit on the floor rather than on chairs. But now, our hip joints have lost the flexibility to squat or even sit in a simple cross-legged position.

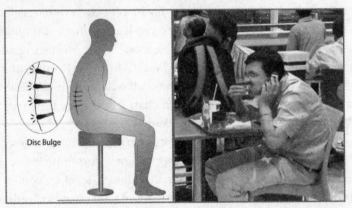

Sitting with a rounded back

It is difficult to sit for prolonged periods on a chair. Our body slouches in a C shape as seen in the figures above. The slouched posture makes the belly muscles completely loose and flabby. Lack of belly tone puts uneven pressure on different parts of the spine, irritates the surrounding nerves and triggers back pain.

This posture also constricts the abdominal organs, which leads to digestive and urinary problems. A slouched posture does not let the diaphragm expand normally, leading to shallow breathing, feeling of exhaustion and other respiratory problems. The muscles from the shoulders down to the knees are completely inert for the duration we sit on a chair.

Craned Head and Neck

With an increase in the number of desk jobs, the head is exercised more than the body. This puts undue strain on the neck muscles to hold up the craning head peering into the computer screen. At the structural level, the head and the neck need support from the body to keep their movements fluid and effortless. However, a rounded back and stooped shoulders with a collapsed chest do not give the neck and the head adequate support. The neck muscles are over strained

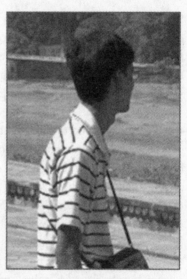

A craned neck and a jutting head

trying to support the head by themselves. The result: the head is either craning forward or hanging down.

Sitting while Driving

A daily commute is now an integral part of our daily routine and driving a car is second nature to many. Long drives seem to be the primary cause of backache. In a moving vehicle, the back is most affected by the constant acceleration, deceleration and swaying from side to side.

Normally, when we are seated on a chair, our feet are placed on the floor to stabilize the lower body. While driving, the constant manipulating of the clutch, the brake and the accelerator does not allow the feet to stabilize the lower body. The car seat is not designed to support the back for a long period of driving and thus increases the chance of back problems. A long-term exposure to the vibrations from driving can also cause backache.

Sleeping Habits

Sleep is an essential factor for a healthy body and mind. A good night's sleep induces a feeling of bliss and is an escape from the trials and tribulations of the day. It is a natural way to restore and reset the body. We are all aware of the association between sleep and emotional well-being, but few of us understand the significance of the position we sleep in. The quality of sleep and the benefits accrued depend on how we sleep.

We spend anywhere between five to eight hours sleeping in our favourite position – about a third of the twenty four hours and a third of our life span! To ignore this significant portion of our lives is a recipe for disaster. Needless to say, it is a good idea to correct any wrongs that we do during our sleeping hours.

Certain sleeping positions actually threaten the natural alignment of our body. They increase the chance of us waking up with a sore back, neck pains and stiffness. We usually blame the mattress or the pillow for the pain and stiffness. However, the fault can more often than not be traced to incorrect sleeping positions.

Sleeping on the Belly

Sleeping with the belly down is never a symmetrical sleeping position. In this position, the head has to turn to one side and this pressurizes the neck. Even the lower back tends to

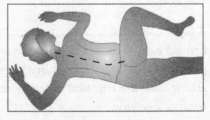

Sleeping on the belly

curve more than its natural turn, to be further pressed into the mattress.

Sleeping on the Side with a Deeply Rounded Back

Most of us sleep on our side in a cuddled up position also known as the foetal position. We are nurtured in the mother's womb in this position. In the pre-natal phase of our lives, every part of the body is supple and springy. As adults, sleeping with a deep curl like a C puts pressure on the spine and its fragile components. Over a period of time, this pressure causes damage.

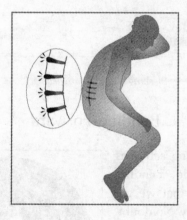

Sleeping on the side with a rounded back

Sleeping on the Side with a Twist at the Waist

Many people with wide hips and broad shoulders sleep on the side out of habit. The waist remains suspended and twists at the parts between the hips and the shoulders. This can lead to muscle imbalance and pain in the lower back. There are some who over-fold the leg on top as compared to the lower one while sleeping on the side. This twists the body at the waist and the back may be stiff on waking up in the morning. Even the head, neck and spine alignment suffers as the body remains twisted and imbalanced.

Sleeping on the Back with a Deeply Arched Lower Back

When persons with a deeply arched lower back sleep on the back, various components of the spine are deprived of adequate blood circulation. The surrounding muscles go into a spasm due to the abnormal curvature of the back. Thus, the muscles of the spine remain tense through the night and are sore on getting up.

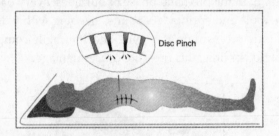

Sleeping on an overarched back

Bending Forward

Of all the routine activities that humans do, bending forward is one that we get wrong frequently. No doubt, most people cannot bend for even a few minutes without pain. The ideal way to bend forward is to use our thigh and abdominal muscles. But most fitness experts do not teach this adequately. It is easier for them to instruct us to stop bending forward than to enlighten us about the correct technique to bend

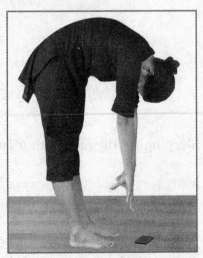

Bending forward

forward. Let's see the two common and incorrect ways in which we bend.

Bending Forward with a Rounded Back

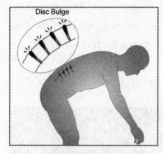

Bending forward with a rounded back

Our general tendency is to bend forward from the waist, with a rounded lower back. Doing this squashes together the front part of the spine, causing premature wear and tear. The compressing action pushes the spinal discs backward and creates a disc bulge. This bulge is likely to squeeze the important nerves that connect at the spine, which may cause pain, tingling sensations and numbness along the pathway of those nerves.

Bending Forward with a Sagged Belly

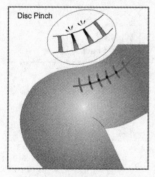

A sagging belly with a disc pinch

A sagged belly is the result of lax muscle tone in the abdomen. When we bend forward, this drooping belly tends to pull the spine down, reduces the muscular support and splints it. Bending forward in this case leads to the spinal discs being pinched together with pain.

The Outcome

A stiff back on waking up, a pulsating lower back, burning discomfort with a tingling sensation in the neck and arms or creaking and clicking of knees – these have become ubiquitous. Someone somewhere is complaining of pain.

Joint pain is not necessarily a function of aging. In this era, it seems people of any age are prone to it. This is alarming news! Does this mean we have to stop standing, walking, sitting, sleeping and bending forward? No; of course, not. The power to relieve ourselves from the pain we suffer is in our own hands. The first step is to identify the cause of the pain, which is what we are on our way to doing here.

Posture-induced pain is caused by wrong habits when we:

Stand	Walk	Sit on a chair	Sleep	Bend forward
With uneven weight on feet	With a dragging gait	With the thighs crossed	On the belly	With a rounded back
With a wide V stance	With a flip-flop gait	With a rounded back	On the side	With a sagging belly
With more weight on one leg	With the heels striking emphatically	With a craned head and neck	With a C back	
With the belly hanging			With an arched back	

Chapter 4

HOW TO TAKE ADVANTAGE OF THIS BOOK?

Good health results from perfect communication between each part of the body and mind.
~ BKS Iyengar

Postural problems are usually a mistake of our making; not of aging. We rarely ever comprehend what we do wrong for these problems to crop up. The 'ignore' approach to our body, while at work and home, is an unconscious act. We conveniently mould our postures to professional demands – a techie's rounded shoulders and protruded head, a beautician's craned neck, a teacher's locked knees, a shopkeeper's arched back from standing for long hours and a couch potato's slouched lower back.

This book is about the powerful effects of developing awareness of our bodies. It is a guide written in a lucid style to enhance the experience of joyful living. It is an attempt to incorporate and interweave, in a practical and illustrative manner, the facts and effects of round-the-clock awareness, safe movements and specific yoga-based practices. It is an attempt to encourage the reader to experience the organic and holistic benefits of yoga to lead a pain-free life.

The fundamentals that constitute the ABC of this book are:

Awareness – accepting our body's limits based on its alignments.

Balance – between flexibility and strength of muscles.

Core – connecting deep.

Awareness

Routine exercise for an hour or two of any type – yoga, walks, gym workouts, athletics, may be an instrument to keep us physically active. However, if the rest of the day is devoid of physical well-being, an hour of physical fitness may prove to be ineffective. Complacency must not allow old bad habits to resurface. It is easy for us to be dragged back to our comfort zones, which was the cause of the problem in the first place. We need to be alert and vigilant to avoid this. To change our destructive pattern of posture and movement, it is essential to maintain a round-the-clock, good postural alignment in our routine activities – YOGA 24 x 7.

Building higher levels of awareness is a technique we need to adopt in conjunction with our modern lifestyle. The seemingly incompatible jet age and the ancient practice of yoga *can* work in tandem to give excellent results for a lifetime. Being aware of oneself is the key to unlocking the benefits of yoga in this modern age.

Self-awareness coupled with yoga creates a dynamic healing process within oneself and leads to a rejuvenated you in mind and body. Let us all salute the great Indian ascetics and masters for preserving the inimitable treasure trove of yoga: Self Awareness!

Balance

A good posture must become a natural and relaxed part of the being. When joints are in alignment with well-toned muscles, it makes for a relaxed body during physical activity. Yoga round the clock is a gentle practice of the yogic principles of alignment for all day-to-day activities.

The traditional approach to pain management is to isolate and exercise individual groups of muscles. When something goes wrong with our musculoskeletal system, we are often directed to exercise the affected muscles, when in fact our body works as an integrated whole. Sustained results can be achieved not by isolating individual muscle groups but by integrating healthy movements and postural patterns for the body, 24 x 7!

Core

The power of the core is unfathomable; it is the point of all physical activity, active and healthy metabolism, inspiration and intuition. Don't we say: I have a gut feeling that...? The core is the temple or the atrium where the body's physical and metaphysical units harmonize on a single plane. It is the core that guides the human body towards better performance, intellectually and physically.

To be aware of the core and to be able to balance its strength and flexibility are of utmost importance. Commonly, the abdomen is said to house the core of our physical body. It is amazing how just a little attention to how we hold the core helps it in holding our body upright and pain-free. Needless to say, this adds to an elegant stance and a radiating personality.

Unlearn and Relearn

Now that we are aware of the importance of posture, it is time to delve deeper into the mechanics of how our body functions, how we deviate from it and how we can fix it effectively and efficiently.

The ensuing chapters are broken into smaller sections for easy understanding. Some information – the techniques to realign the body – may be found to be subtly repetitive to drive home the important points. These are what we like to call the 'Instant Relief Mantras'. These mantras show up often as:

- they are of utmost importance;

- each alignment or postural correction they are mentioned for would be incomplete without them;

- and most important, we tend to forget them and need repeated reminders.

The sections flow as follows:

Recognize

To recognize is the foundation of a good posture. In this section, we will try to comprehensively understand the three basic principles of proper posture – Awareness, Balance and Core. This section is an attempt at improving our health and attitude by just being aware of our body. This awareness cannot come about without knowing how nature has designed us and what goes wrong because we are not aware. We then elaborate on how an involved core is the prerequisite of a good posture.

Realign

The next step is to address the problems discovered and realign the body to its correct position. This section assists in finding the problems – joint and muscle imbalances and their solutions. Beginning at the feet, the understanding of the problems and their solutions moves upward to the head. It covers all the major joints; knees, lower back, upper back, shoulders and neck – and their functions.

Along with each of these important joints, this section contains descriptions of the human physical structure in absolute layman terms. This knowledge helps us understand and appreciate the way our body is meant to function. Once we are aware of our body structure, the easy pointers in the book help self-assess our posture for each particular joint. This section also has observations about the common ways in which these postures go wrong.

The section ends with prescriptions to get the postures right, to reduce, if not to get rid of, pains and aches. It thus educates the reader to gain scientific knowledge as well as an inner knowledge that helps create harmony on the inside and an aura of peace and dignity on the outside.

Reunite

Here, the awareness is reinforced with practical and simple techniques to re-establish natural and healthy postural and movement patterns. The focus is on training and maintaining a body free from disabling pain. Constant self-awareness utilizes body movement to the optimum. A single alignment correction creates a ripple effect in the body by improving other related joint alignments. We take a holistic look at how we can bring mindfulness to our body as a whole in day-to-day activities like standing, sitting, walking, driving, sleeping and so on. Apply these concepts for an awesome makeover!

The content in this book does not replace expert, medical advice (Refer to Page 56, Chapter 7 for details on when it is important to seek medical advice). When in pain, do value medical advice, but do not stop at short-term fixes. Remember, life is a learning process and we are sure this book will help resolve issues.

It is never too late to undo wrong habits and replace them with new and helpful ones. The time taken to start reaping the benefits of practice differs from person to person. Contrary to common belief, once the key principles have been imbibed, the techniques put minimal demands on time. Mundane, regular physical activities acquire a refreshing hue and become safe to perform. Let us inculcate the habit of awareness and learn to honour our body's wisdom. Awareness reveals to us a whole new fascinating world. A positive attitude should go a long way in making progress.

Through this book, I share with joy, the art of enhancing the rich life forces to optimal capacity. Best wishes for an exhilarating experience.

Section II

RECOGNIZE

It requires a very unusual mind to undertake the analysis of the obvious.
~ Alfred North Whitehead

Chapter 5

BALANCED MUSCLES

Unless some misfortune has made it impossible,
everyone can have good posture.
~ Loretta Young

Kabir, *an upcoming lawyer, has to be a part of countless meetings. Being a voracious reader, his after work hours are spent reading, curled up in bed. He knows he has a sedentary lifestyle and therefore religiously works out for 90 minutes every day. In spite of the workout, Kabir suffers from lower back and neck pains. The reason – bad postural habits.*

Exercises meant to strengthen the core muscles prove to be ineffective if the posture is imbalanced. In fact, the benefits of a proper workout are washed out due to lack of awareness of our body alignment. What is needed is to be sensitive to the posture and the baseline tone in muscles while following the techniques of proper maintenance of bone and joint alignment to the core.

Assess Your Alignment

Different parts of our body need to be in line with one other for our body to be properly aligned. Just as an edifice needs beams and pillars in perfect alignment for a strong foundation, our bones and joints too need proper symmetry, both vertically and horizontally. This helps in keeping the body from leaning forward or backward, or tilting to any side. It also ensures good functioning, minimal wear and tear and prevention of loss of energy.

Vertical Alignment

The human body is seen to be vertically aligned when the bones of the body are placed over one another in line with gravity. If the head is habitually protruded, which is quite common, it takes unusual effort for the muscles of the neck to hold it in that position.

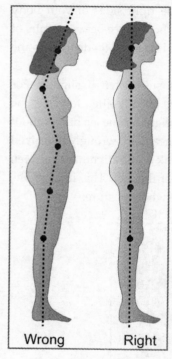

Wrong   Right

Vertical alignment of joints

The muscles eventually over-strain and fatigue because they are in a state of constant contraction or 'spasm'. A chronic hunch over the office table spoils the alignment of the bones of the spine, leading to tension in the upper back and the neck.

The **plumb-line technique** is a simple method to understand the vertical alignment of different body parts with respect to each other. Imagine a string tied from the crown of your head, down to the feet. This is referred to as the plumb-line. In an ideal situation, when you look at it from the side, it will go over the ear, the shoulder, the hip and the centre of the knee, and end just in front of the ankle. From the front, the imaginary line passes over the centre of the back of the head, over every vertebra, the cleft of the buttocks, midway between the two knees and midway between the heels. This is the blueprint of our body's map. The following conclusions can be drawn:

- If the head and the shoulder are ahead of this line, then it is the forward head position. This may be accompanied by an increased upper back hump.

- If the centre of the knee is behind the line, then the knees are locked, that is, they are hyper-extended or over-straightened. If the knees are over-bent, the centre is ahead of this line.

Horizontal Alignment

The balance between the left and the right sides of your body defines its horizontal alignment. It is the balance between pairs of bones, like shoulders, hips, knees and heels, at 90 degrees to the plumb-line.

Almost all of us slump to one side, even if slightly. For example, shoulders of a bike rider are usually tilted towards one side. Similarly, standing with more weight on one leg brings about misaligned knees. This can lead to knee pain, wrongly perceived as arthritis. The arches of the feet speak of the alignment between the bones of the ankle and the rest of the feet. This impacts the way we stand and walk and thus the whole posture.

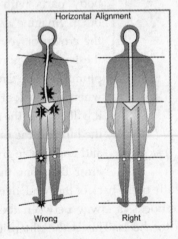

Horizontal alignment of joints

Role of Muscles in Maintaining Alignment

The bones and the joints of the body work in tandem with the muscles to maintain the alignment of the body and to perform any activity. The best teamwork and symbiotic relationships are observed in the human body itself. Muscles play a pivotal role in aligning the bones with each other to maintain good posture and to allow free and efficient movements of different joints. Different groups of muscles are assigned to the skeleton at various vantage points. These hold the body upright against gravity and make movement possible.

Functionally, the muscles in the body can be understood as:

Mobilizing Muscles or Muscles for Movement at Joints – Muscles at joints in the body function in pairs and form a muscle group. For every muscle present in front of a joint, there is a corresponding muscle behind that joint. For example, muscles on the front and behind your upper arm (that make shoulder and elbow movements possible) or the muscle groups on the front part of your thigh and behind (that make hip and knee movements possible).

To move a body part, the muscle at the front of the joint contracts, while the one behind stretches. At the same joint, to make a converse movement, the muscle behind contracts and the one at the front stretches. For example, when you straighten your leg at the knee, the front part of the thigh muscle (quadriceps) contracts, while the one behind (hamstrings) stretches. On the other hand, when you bend the leg at the knee, the front part of the thigh muscle stretches, while the one behind contracts. A smooth movement of the body involves the co-ordination of the muscles.

Muscles have to be both strong and flexible to enable such movement. Proper alignment is possible with the help of healthy muscles working in sync with each other.

Stabilizing Muscles or Muscles for Stability and Core Strength – Stabilizing muscles do the tasks of keeping us erect and connecting the spine – the central axis of the body – to the arms and the legs. The natural tone of these muscles is crucial for the stability of our posture and movements. The luxury that modern technology grants us has weakened our core strength to a considerable extent. The new age life increasingly revolves around apparel, furniture and gadgets that require us to stand, sit and move in ways that weaken our core.

Root Cause of Pain: Imbalanced Muscles of Mobility

Our muscles are the primary shock absorbers of the body and need to work in harmony to keep the joints stress-free and mobile, without friction. This requires optimum use of the muscles at all times. Strength and flexibility of an entire muscle group is necessary for good joint movement. Regrettably, this balance is rarely preserved. We end up either underusing or overusing our muscles.

All of us have at some time experienced tightness in muscles. When we quit walking and exercising for a few months or even weeks, the result is muscle rigidity. The correct amount of contracting and stretching of muscles regularly keeps them in good shape and condition.

Muscles need to be gently worked to their optimum level, or they lose their elasticity to become lax and weak. This weakness of the muscles is compensated by the overuse of adjacent muscles, which gradually start tightening. The tightened muscles in turn overpower the opposing weak muscles to weaken them further. This leads to a chain of imbalances, inevitably followed by pain and suffering.

Overused Muscles

If one of the muscles in the pair – front or back, right or left – is overused, it gets tighter than its partner. This happens to all of us and a common example of this is tight hamstrings – the muscles behind the thigh that extend up to the knee. These muscles are in a constant state of contraction when we sit for long hours.

Overused muscles shorten and tighten over time, and create problems. When the hamstring muscles tighten and shorten, straightening the knee becomes difficult, even for people who are slim and have shapely figures. To reinstate the balance, the overused muscles need calculated stretches to lengthen them appropriately.

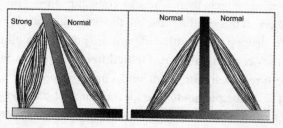

Misalignment of overused muscles in comparison to their natural alignment

Underused Muscles

Underdeveloped or underused muscles lose their normal tone and become flabby, soft and atrophied. To understand, let's see how the quadriceps muscle is affected due to sitting on the chair for several hours at a stretch.

Our legs are folded when we sit on a chair. In this position, the quadriceps, or the muscles in front of the thigh, are in a state of constant relaxation. This makes them weak as they are not used as much as the hamstrings, or the muscles at the back of the thigh, are. To balance the muscle tone of the quadriceps, we need to reactivate and strengthen them by stretching them.

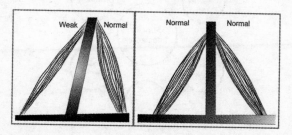

Misalignment of underused muscles in comparison to their natural alignment

Constant Tug-of-War

The under and overuse of muscles in a muscle group results in a constant of tug-of-war among the muscles. The outcome of this disharmony is pain.

Imbalanced muscles pull at our bones and joints to cause displacement, which then leads to constant stress and uneven pressure on all three – the muscles, the bones and the joints. This is akin to driving a car with different air pressure in all the four tyres. If the car continues to run with different air pressure in each tyre, the tyres wear out faster and engine depreciation sets in earlier. This principle holds true for the human body too!

The synchronization among muscles determines the condition of the joints. It determines whether the joints are put through the stress, the strain or the grinding that occurs in and around the joint. Even a marginal misalignment of the muscles is enough to drastically alter the tension inside the joint. If the muscles on one side are stronger than their counterparts on the other side, the joint either slightly tilts or rotates, getting harmed as the bones move away from their natural axis.

Poor alignment compounds the stress and the strain on the joints and the muscles. The muscles supporting the bones and the joints are exerted beyond their natural capacities, forcing them to carry more weight and lose elasticity.

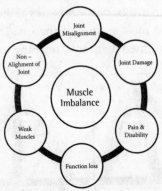

Vicious cycle of muscle imbalance

So then, what exactly is good posture?

Good posture involves maintaining the body in:

- proper vertical alignment.
- proper horizontal alignment.

A correct posture indicates:

- strong and supple muscles which keep bones and joints in the correct alignment;
- minimal stress on the joints;
- that joints do not get fixated in abnormal positions;
- that muscles are used efficiently, allowing the body to conserve energy and preventing fatigue;
- increased metabolism to burn more calories;
- an attractive personality boosted by self-confidence.

How to Maintain Alignment

Identify Safe Middle Range of Joint Position and Movement

Each muscle has an optimal length and angle where it works at its best. At this length and angle, it is neither overstretched nor over-contracted. Similarly, every joint has an optimal middle range of movement where it is neither over-bent, nor too open. Keeping a joint within its optimal middle range allows the muscles around it to operate at their optimal length. Muscles are strongest at this length, with least likelihood of damage and fatigue.

Exercise Muscles

Muscles on both sides of the middle range should be exercised for the purpose of strengthening and stretching them, so that they can handle some deviations from the norm without getting harmed.

Tone Core

Abdominal muscles, also aptly referred to as the core, are stabilizing muscles that play a pivotal role in maintaining a good posture. The topic of the right amount of tone in the core will be frequently brought up in the subsequent chapters. Yet its importance cannot be emphasized enough. A toned core, apart from being the fulcrum of good health, lends a slimming effect to the body and shows as a beaming, energized personality.

A sedentary lifestyle, combined with stress, fears and anxieties, subjects the muscles to uncomfortable spasms and tightness. A stressful frame of mind, coupled with lack of exercise, ultimately creates muscle disharmony. The problem is further compounded by advancing age as the muscles become weaker and less resilient. The body starts bending closer to the ground which lowers the center of gravity. To avoid these problems, we must consciously start to invest time and effort early on in our lives.

We maltreat our body, mostly unknowingly. If we were better informed about the consequences, we would certainly be precautious. However, it is never too late. The ensuing chapters will share simple steps to a good posture and pain-free living, ranging from insightful details on a strong core to the treatment of the major pain zones in the body.

Chapter 6

STABILITY OF THE CORE

Make your belly your best friend.
~ Osho

Tuck your tummy in slightly, hold it there and look in the mirror; you cannot help gush over this metamorphosis! If this short-lived change can be such a rewarding experience, imagine what it would be like if you could make this 'wow look' a lifetime possession? Feel triumphant for the lifelong gift you are about to give yourself: Great posture, regal carriage, confident composure, classic appearance, booming self-confidence and much more.

How we handle our core directly reflects on our posture and mental attitude. Bad posture signifies insecurity, diffidence and, worst of all, an inferiority complex. Good posture symbolises poise, good body shape and natural ease. Posture is not about stiff attention but about a state of poised comfort.

At the physical level, core is the fulcrum on which the body mechanism rests. A toned core provides us strength and stability that translates into a pleasing personality. Activating the core muscles should be a priority since most of us tend to have a weak core. The combination of correct posture and a toned core can make us look 2-5 kg slimmer and several inches taller.

At the energy level, breathing correctly sustains the oxygen levels required to remain energetic in body and spirit. Employing the correct technique of deep breathing, utilizing the abdominal muscles and the diaphragm, increases the oxygen flow in the system. Deep breathing also tones the pelvic floor muscles.

Structure

To activate the magic of a toned core, let's begin by understanding its structure. The core is situated in the region below the chest and above the pelvis. To understand its structure, think of a house as similar to the body, where the:

1. Diaphragm is the ceiling.
2. Abdominal muscles (abs) are the front wall.
3. Hip muscles (gluts) and the deep lower back muscles are the back wall.

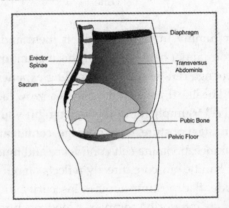

Core abdominal muscles

All the abdominal organs – liver, stomach, intestines, kidneys, important endocrine glands, major nerve junctions – live and breathe in this house. To keep the structure intact, all the muscles need to be working correctly and in tandem.

Diaphragm

The diaphragm is a large, parachute-shaped muscle that moves with each breath. It is connected to the lower six ribs and the last six vertebrae of the thoracic spine (the thoracic spine has 12 vertebrae, all of which attach to the ribs). The diaphragm is also attached to the front side of many lumbar region (lower back) bones. Therefore, anything that restricts the movement of the diaphragm affects the spine.

The diaphragm plays a primary role in breathing. It expands the breathing space while inhaling and contracts it while exhaling. Most of the sensations we feel when we inhale come from the outward expansion of the belly and the lower ribs, a movement created by the action of the diaphragm.

Abdominal Muscles (Abs)

The abdominal muscles create a band-like support for the core. The abs, along with the lower back muscles, weave a strong natural corset around the all-important lower spine. Abdominal muscles are multi-layered and form the front part of the corset.

i. Outer Corset

The outer corset of the abs is a superficial layer of muscles popularly known as the six pack abs. This layer forms the upper layer of the abdomen's wall in the front. The oblique abdominal muscles that flank the waist also integrate with these muscles to make up the outer corset.

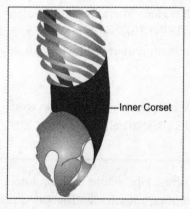

Inner corset or transversus abdominis

ii.   Inner Corset

The transversus abdominis (TA) muscle is a broad horizontal sheet of muscle that lies deep beneath the outer corset. It forms a protective wrap around the abdominal organs and is attached not only to the spine at the back but also to the lower ribs and the pelvis in the front. The contraction of TA flattens and compresses the abdominal space. The oblique abdominal muscles integrate with the TA muscle to further strengthen the core.

Hip Muscles (Gluts)

The buttock or the hip muscles play a crucial role in providing support to the core from the back. The weakness of the gluts is rampant due to our chair-bound culture, where we do not need to use them. This central weakness affects the health of the lower back and the legs.

Macho or Poncho – Where is the in-between?

'Surf Board' Abs: We have bought into the notion that stiff abs are the hallmark of a strong core. On the one hand, we have crunch-obsessed fitness buffs with power-packed muscles – the surf board abs! Unfortunately, these macho abs aren't necessarily the best. If done wrong, crunches can restrict breathing, causing all sorts of disharmony in the body.

Loose Bellies: On the other hand, we have people who are victims of a sedentary, chair-bound lifestyle. Their abs are lost in folds of fat where no tricks of fashion can camouflage the reality. The fat cells seem to have a special affinity to the belt region, where they accumulate to give birth to a poncho belly! This bulge grows slowly and steadily, ruling the midriff region until we wake up to start the battle of the core.

Between these two extremes, there is an in-between. The keyword here, like for everything else in life, is: Balance!

Weak Core: A Reality

In the past, man was physically active in farms and at home, and thus had strong muscles with good core strength. Today, our comfort-driven lifestyle has made our core weak. It is our core that is our essence; not the 'six pack abs'. A strong core comprises toned postural muscles combined with the all-important healthy abdominal breathing. A weak core shows up as:

› Toneless abdomen or an over-tight abdomen
› Rounded upper back
› Shallow breathing
› Weakened metabolism
› Hormonal imbalances
› Mental instabilities

Do It Right – Navel in, but Gently

A healthy baseline tone in the muscles is a pre-requisite for stable posture and movements. The action of the inner corset or the TA is fundamental to the stabilization of posture. A strong central support makes it possible to let go of the compensatory tension we carry in different parts of the body. A harmonious balance is achieved when the inner corset gives continuous support and the outer corset helps build strength and movement.

A healthy core tone is not the result of sporadic exercise. Constant awareness of baseline tone is essential, be it while standing, sitting or moving. The TA should be mildly contracted to recover the lost tone. This should not, however, be confused with sucking in the abdomen. Rigid and statue-like demeanour by sucking the belly in is not building core tone, which can, in fact, be detrimental as it constricts breathing.

Experience the magic instead by pulling in the navel by just half an inch. Doing so contributes to only about 5-10% contraction of the TA muscles, which is sufficient to support the lower back and prevent problems.

• Sit straight and simply observe your natural breaths.

• Now, pull the navel in by just half an inch; let it stay there comfortably.

• If you over-tighten the navel, you will begin to hold your breaths. This should be corrected immediately by relaxing the navel and trying a gentler squeeze again.

Squeezing your navel in this manner renders deep breathing, thus reinvigorating your mind and body. The flow of energy is remarkable. Remember to observe and apply this simple technique as often as possible to get the best out of breathing. The beauty of this technique is that you can practise this anywhere, anytime with absolute ease. It has amazing effects and, most of all, it is absolutely free!

Benefits of using the inner corset:

- Stretches the spine, while being safe and natural.
- Helps stabilize the spine.
- Protects the spine during acts of compression, distortion and high impact.
- Provides stability for better arm and leg functioning.
- Tones the lower abdomen and raises the height by at least half an inch.
- Fires up the metabolic rate.

An active, round-the-clock metabolism is a dream for many of us for its weight management advantages. While it looks difficult to achieve an active metabolism, postural corrections is often all it takes to reach there. In fact, by merely pulling in our navel slightly, we can awaken the sleeping metabolism. This is one of the best kept secrets to a strong and refined metabolism!

So, whether you are leaning on the kitchen platform, slouching in your office chair, lifting objects from the floor or carrying weights – just hum this TA tone mantra: *Navel in!*

Do It Right – The Hip Clench

You can stand, sit or lie down to do this practice. In fact, you can do it even as you walk!

- As you exhale, gently pull the belly in.

- Clench the hip region, gently engaging the muscles of the region. This will help bring the pelvis in the neutral position and reduce the extra arch at the lower back.

- Hold this gentle squeeze position for a comfortable period of time.

Do It Right – Breathe Out, Belly In. Breathe In, Belly Out

Diaphragmatic breaths involve breathing to the belly, the ribs and the lower back. This automatically corrects chronic chest breathing and often relieves backaches instantly. To be pain-free, you have to keep the spinal muscles healthy, balanced and well-toned, all enthusiastically. An easy way to start breathing right is while lying down in bed before falling asleep.

- Lie down on our back.

- Place your hands on your belly.

- Gently bring your focus to your breaths.

- Contract the navel area as you exhale. Feel the navel move in towards the spine as the lower back lengthens.

As you inhale, your diaphragm will contract and push down. The belly will bulge out gently under your hands. This upward and outward expansion indicates that the abdominal organs have released and are lengthening. The belly should rise before the chest does. Simply let everything relax when you exhale.

Each time you take a complete breath, you tone your abdominal muscles. Practice the same belly, ribs and lower back inhalation while sitting or standing. The more often you practice, the stronger the diaphragm's motor patterns grow. Classic places to practice are while waiting at stoplights, during commercial breaks and whenever you feel stressed. Once you are attuned to breathing right, the technique can be attempted during all day-to-day activities.

Benefits of Deep Breathing

On an average, we breathe 20,000 times a day. Despite that, the power of breathing is underestimated by most people.

Studies have shown that sedentary conveniences hinder our calorie loss by about 800 calories. Since most of us tend to be shallow breathers, we utilize a mere 25% of the oxygen capacity of our lungs. Deep breathing increases the capacity of the lungs by 75%, which in turn maximizes the body's calorie-burning ability. Studies reveal that with simple, deep breathing, we can burn off 140% more calories than by exercising on a stationary bike. Conscious deep breathing practice for just 30 minutes a day burns 350 calories. Moreover, improving quality of breaths boosts the immune system.

Effective breathing requires good postural habits and a mild baseline tone in our abdominal muscles. Just sitting straight and energising the lower belly by pulling the navel in by a mere half inch improves our breaths naturally and remarkably.

Enduring changes come about only with a paradigm shift in attitude – when we become enlightened about ourselves. Pay attention to your breathing and the core; they will in turn take care of all else. This is an amazing journey of self-exploration. Get ready to conquer the best within you!

Chapter 7

PRINCIPLES OF SAFE YOGA PRACTICES

The man who has no inner life is the slave of
his surroundings.
~ Henri F Amiel

Yoga is acknowledged as remedy only when practised with caution. The essence of practising yoga is to preserve and restore the natural space between bones, with strong and supple support of surrounding muscles and ligaments.

Yoga: Your Own Great Awareness

When yoga postures are done with a 'just get it over' attitude, the practice of yoga can be chaotic and muddled and does not deliver the intended results. Some yoga practitioners are known to perform asanas while watching TV or movies. This is erroneous as yoga is a beautiful blend of the mind and the body. The practice of yogasanas goes beyond a mere mechanical performance of physical exercises; it involves the mind to liberate the body from aches and pains.

Yoga Is Flexibility Based on Strength

Some incredibly flexible people are prone to backaches and injuries. To illustrate the point, let me share a personal experience. At an international yoga conference that I attended in Hong Kong, there were participants from the Far East – Singapore, Korea, Thailand and, of course, Hong Kong. Genetically, people from the

Far East are known to be blessed with a flexible body. They can perform complex yoga postures with absolute ease. Yet, they were at a workshop on 'Yoga for Backache'. I could not believe this, but it was an eye-opener.

I realized that their natural tendency to overdo while performing asanas probably destabilized the joints with subsequent, irrational wear and tear. Over-extending our limits can be harmful even while practising asana.

Yoga Is Not a 'One Size Fits All' Solution

Each person has their own body frame, lifestyle habits, level of flexibility and strength. Yoga practices need to be adapted to a person's individual capacity with the help of bolsters, cushions, chairs, etc.; the selection of the practices themselves varies from person to person. Give a deep thought before selecting a yoga master; he or she must have mastery of the human structure combined with an intuitive spirit to heal.

Yoga Is Different for Men and Women

Yogasanas were invented many centuries ago for the benefit of men. The male of the species has a stronger muscular structure due to the inherent hormonal structure. Besides, a rigid lifestyle with little multi-tasking has led men to have stiff bodies and tight joints. So, their asanas revolved around stretching exercises, using props like ropes and belts to loosen the joints. Women on the other hand were not considered for yogasanas. Hormonally, women have weaker muscles than men. Also, their muscles tend to lose their tone with advancing age and menopause, making them hyper-flexible at the joints as compared to men.

Today, since women practice asanas more than men, the practices need to be adapted to suit the requirements of more and more women. They require more strengthening exercises so they can use their own muscles to hold a posture without the need for props.

Yoga Is Not Doing Only Difficult Postures

People equate yoga with difficult postures and this intimidates many. In its purest forms, yoga makes you know and understand yourself better. There are plenty of simple yogic practices that can be applied 24 x 7. Coupled with scientific knowledge, the power of yoga can enable us to become wiser about our body. Regular practice, under a knowledgeable teacher, ushers in remarkable benefits. You learn to stretch and lengthen the spine gently, lift the body, and realign the head and the neck the way nature meant it. This creates space for the joints to perform their functions, which otherwise get wedged incorrectly due to constraints brought by wrong postures.

First, Do No Harm

It is crucial to avoid common yoga mistakes that can result in injury. When you follow classical yoga guidelines, you are encouraged to seek positions in which you continually experience your body to be comfortable and steady – *sthiram sukham aasanam*.

If at any point, you feel a given posture/practice initiates pain or makes an existing one worse, you are advised to stop the practice immediately and seek medical help for your ailment.

'How We Do' Is More Important Than 'What We Do'

Yoga is all about being constantly mindful of how you are doing it and feeling the positive effects on the body. The awareness that comes with such practices has to be with us round the clock. The following points should be kept in mind.

Postures with Alignment

There should be optimal aligning of bones, supported with strong balanced muscles to prevent wear and tear of joints. Each posture prescribed is described with detailed alignments. Be very careful to follow the alignments.

Strength over Flexibility

Flexibility that cannot be supported by strength should not be aimed for. Even if you are extremely flexible, you may not have the muscle strength to get into certain postures and may end up injuring yourself.

Breathe

When we push too hard while exercising, we tend to hold our breathing. This brings in rigidity rather than stability, and stiffness rather than suppleness. There is also an increased risk of injury.

Less Is More

Never overdo or go beyond the range of safe movements. Progress slowly and steadily; motivate yourself as you move from success to success. Be generous to yourself by moving within your personal pain-free range.

Effortless Effort

Practising yoga has to be as effortless as possible. It requires you to be aware of what is going on in the body so you can make minute changes as per the demands of the body. Make sure that you are relaxed and then proceed to:

- Connect awareness to the spine by engaging your inner core and straightening the back.
- Facilitate movement at the largest joints first – hips and shoulders.
- Maintain core stability.

- Make sure that the movements are optimal at all joints.

- Maintain a balance between strength and suppleness and stability and comfort in the final pose.

- Breathe correctly throughout a pose.

Programming Your Practice Protocol

We are now gearing up to dive deep into understanding our bodies. We will begin by knowing the structure of important joints. We will then make observations regarding how we deviate from what is normal and finally move on to simple practices that can lead us to better postures.

For each joint, a separate chapter has been dedicated detailing postures that can be practised to help with any pain in the region. Do not let the number of practices overwhelm you. You certainly do not have to do them all. Do as much as you can and reap the benefits.

- You can set up a routine where you do a different set of practices every day, specific to your body type and ailment.

- When pressed for time, you can reduce the number of practices. Try not to skip the practices altogether. Like many things in life, something is certainly better than nothing.

- Reduce the number of times you practice a posture rather than reducing the duration for which you hold the posture. For example, it is recommended that you do a certain practice five times and hold the pose for ten seconds. If you are short of time, do it only twice, but do hold the pose for ten seconds each, instead of doing it five times while holding the pose for two seconds each.

Finally, remember that these are very generic practices. Each body is different. I have tried to address issues that people with different body types face. It is for you to pick up practices that go with your body type.

When Should You See a Doctor?

When in doubt, seek professional medical advice. Make sure you see a doctor especially when:

- The pain is due to a fall or an accident.
- There is a line of shooting pain from the back and the hips along the length of one leg.
- There is a line of shooting pain from the neck along the arm.
- The pain is sharp and stabbing, such that it disables you.
- There is numbness or tingling.
- There is weakness in the feet and the leg or a loss of holding power in the hands.
- The exercises are initiating pain which sustains even after the exercise is over.
- The exercises are not helping you.

Section III

REALIGN

What is necessary to change a person is to change his awareness of himself.
~ Abraham H. Maslow

If anything is sacred, the human body is sacred.
~ Walt Whitman

Chapter 8

FOUNDATION FIRST – OUR FEET

Think of the magic of the foot, comparatively small, upon which your whole weight rests. It is a miracle.
~ Martha Graham

Want long-term health insurance without premiums? Invest right away in your feet! Lovingly express gratitude to them for the huge task they perform all through your life. Pamper your feet, for they need as much attention as the face. Feet are the foundation of a good posture, good health and overall well-being.

Despite their relatively small size, our feet are completely responsible for our upright posture and movement. We are oblivious to just how much our feet take the brunt of our body weight, more so in case of obesity. Amazingly, the Indian tradition of touching elders' feet for blessings is also an expression of respect for these invaluable structures.

Structure

Each foot has 26 bones, 32 joints and 38 muscles; the numbers may not seem impressive, but the architecture is mind-boggling. Our humble salutations to the master! Observe this complex structure; see how harmoniously toes, soles, ankles, arches and heels – function, generating intricate, flexible movements with great ease.

To endure rugged movements and bear weight, the bones of our feet are structured with three arches, two longitudinal arches and one horizontal arch. Ligaments and muscles present in the feet support the arches and stabilize the bones.

Longitudinal Arch: The inner longitudinal arch runs from the bottom of the ankle through to the first three toes. The outer longitudinal arch spans from the heels to the fourth and the fifth toes.

Horizontal Arch: The horizontal arch runs through the mounds of the feet in a horizontal plane.

Well-structured arches are a mark of proper alignment and facilitate correct use of feet and ankles. Their suppleness lends our feet a natural spring-like effect and promotes shock absorption. The arches also provide strength and flexibility when we stand or are in motion. When any of these arches loses its structural equilibrium, pain surfaces. This pain is not restricted to the foot, but is transmitted to the legs, the hips and the lower back as well. It is worthwhile to remember that a weak arch can impact the entire body's alignment.

Issues related to arches have increased as we hardly walk barefoot on uneven surfaces these days. As a result of walking on smooth roads and using wrong footwear, deeper muscles which support the arches remain underused and weaken with time. Consequently, the arches lose their ability to work in cohesion, and sometimes lead to flat feet and heel spurs.

Self-Assessment

The way we place our feet on the ground has a direct impact on our legs and knees. We will discuss common postural habits and how they cause misalignments, and provide a list of corrections later on in the chapter. Before that, just answer the following questions.

Where do toes and mounds point? Stand barefoot on a flat surface in front of a full length mirror. Imagine that you are standing in the middle of a clock with your toes facing the number 12. Look at your feet in the mirror and see where the great toes are pointing – away from the midline, parallel to each other or inward?

Toes and ankles:

- Does the big toe pull inward towards the other toes?

- Are the toes bent and curled, or straight?

- Are the ankles rolled in, rolled out or centrally placed?

Feel the body weight:

- Does one foot bear more weight than the other?

- Where is the pressure felt more – the heels or the mounds of the toes?

- Where is weight borne more – the outer or the inner edges of the feet?

Arch of the feet: Wet your feet. Step on a dark surface. Look at the points of contact between your feet and the floor. They will leave wet impressions and enable us to assess the arch.

- Normal arch: You have normal arch feet if the connecting strip between the toes and the heels is about half the width of respective feet.

- High arch: You have high arch feet if the outline of the toes and the balls of the feet are connected with the heel by a very thin strip.

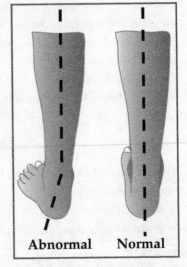

Abnormal   Normal

Abnormal and normal positioning of toes and ankles

- Flat feet: If the connecting strip between your toes and heels is more than half the width of the respective feet or if the entire outline of the foot shows, you have flat feet.

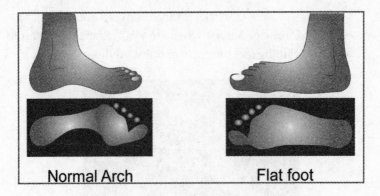

Normal Arch   Flat foot

Impressions made by a normal arch foot and a flat foot

Assess your walk: Walk a few steps with complete awareness. Read the questions below and then walk a few more steps with the intention of finding your answers to these questions.

• Where do the heels meet the ground – at the centre, inner or outer edges of the heels?

• Is the impact on both the heels equal?

• Do you actively place your toes down first with each step and push off from the toes to take the next step? Or is it just a passive rollover action with the heel touching the ground first?

• Do your buttocks or the hip muscles have some tone when the heel strikes the ground?

• After you place your leg on the floor, does the knee of that leg push behind into a locked position? (Locked knee means the knee over-straightens.)

Common Observations

Let's quickly revisit the common postures that the legs assume when we walk or stand.

Feet Placed Like a V: The two feet are significantly turned outward when we stand or walk (the distance between both sets of toes is more than the distance between both heels). This creates a torque or a twist when we walk, as the legs want to go ahead but the feet move in an outward direction.

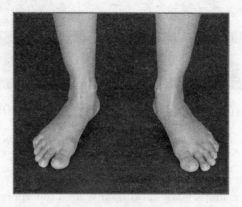

Wide V standing posture

Unequal Weight Distribution: Most of us stand on only a part of a foot. Some people put more weight on the outer edges of our feet, so that the heels and the inner edges of the feet do not share in the distribution of the weight. On the contrary, flat-footed people tend to stand on the inner edges of their feet. The unequal weight distribution disturbs the relationship between and the stability of the ankle, the knee and the hip joints.

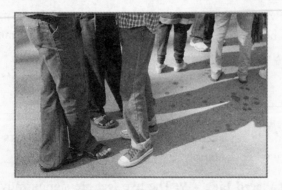

Unequal weight distribution

Rolling on the Ankles: The unequal and disproportionate spread of weight between the two edges of a foot tends to roll the ankles. People with flat feet and low arches tend to have ankles that collapse inward. This increases the load borne by the inside of the knees. On the other hand, people with high arches roll the weight on the outside of the foot to rotate the leg bones outward, which affects the outer side of their knees.

Faulty Walking and Feet Abuse: When a foot falls on the floor without being properly aligned with the ground, there is an excessive foot roll. The leg, the ankle and the respective knee turn and collapse sideways, followed by rapid forceful changes in the leg alignment. This grinds the bones at the joints.

Toes have shock absorbers and are designed to initiate movement. However, we do not adequately push off from the toes when we walk, due to which they lose their normal shape. And since, in doing so we leave the task of moving the body forward to the knees, the knees end up getting deranged.

The good news is that none of the problems arising out of bad postures are permanent. Our awareness about the way our feet should behave when we walk or stand can free us of present and future problems. We discuss this later on in the chapter.

Structural Alterations

It is said that a person can be judged on personal care from the way they take care of their feet. Unfortunately, we pay our feet minimal attention, especially when it comes to their functional structure.

Flat Feet: As is often believed, flat feet are not always a birth defect. Like I mentioned before, flat feet may be caused by weak, collapsing arches – an outcome of the fact that we no longer walk barefoot. With fallen arches, the inner edges of the soles come closer to the floor. This makes the weight of the body concentrate on the inner edges, instead of being spread evenly on the feet, so that the shock absorption function of the feet gets disturbed and the impact travels beyond the knees.

Special footwear can mechanically lift the arches, but real benefits come with the use of muscles via corrective exercises. Simple exercises help awaken the sleeping muscles and rebuild the healthy curvatures of the feet.

Footwear Matters: The right footwear should support the arches not just structurally but functionally too. The feet muscles should get adequately stretched and worked so that the body weight gets evenly distributed on the weight-bearing points of the feet.

i.   **High Heels:** Wedges, stilettos or other kinds of high heels alter the structural position of the heel in relation to the rest of the foot. This disturbs the balance between the different weight-bearing joints in many ways.

   The foot slides to the front of the shoe, adding unwanted pressure on the mounds of the toes. The ankle tendon at the end of the calf muscle gets shortened, causing the muscles in front of the ankle to stretch and weaken, and the feet to experience pain and fatigue.

   High heels cause an unreasonable tilt in the ankle. In order to avoid a fall, all other joints are forced to adapt. The price of this adjustment is muscle stiffness, painful feet and aching joints, which span into the lower back.

   For women with musculoskeletal dys-function, high heels are an invite to big trouble.

ii. **Narrow Pointed Shoes:** Such shoes squeeze the toes, disturb the arches and make them flatter. A shift in the weight-bearing axis triggers a vicious cycle that leads to degeneration. The damage is not localized to the feet, and extends to the ankles, the knees, the hips and the back too because the muscles in these parts are all connected and depend on one another for their well-being.

Do It Right – Stand Smart

One of the most useful ways to correct discomfort experienced when standing, is to pay attention to the feet. By becoming conscious of the placement of our feet on the ground, we can control the balance of the entire body. A balance between the outer and the inner arches and between the toe mounds and the heels is the foundation of a stable stance and a graceful walk. Knee pain and spinal disorders too improve frequently with balanced feet.

Parallel Feet: When the two feet are parallel to each other, the weight-bearing axis of the body is aligned, so that there is minimal stress to the joints. This alignment can be further fine-tuned by turning the toes slightly in, by just half an inch, such that the outer edges of the two feet are parallel to each other. This has beneficial effects on the knees, as it prevents them from locking. To develop the habit of standing with your feet parallel to each other, you can begin by standing on a mat and aligning the outer edges of your feet with the outline of mat.

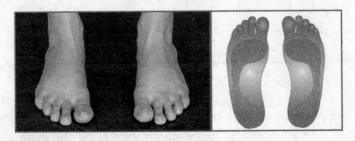

Parallel feet

Hip-Width Distance between the Two Feet: Hip-width distance is understood as the widest part of our visible hip region. However, from a healthy alignment point of view, the hip-width distance is the distance between the hip joints, which are more towards the midline of the body. A good approximation of this distance is the distance between our two ears. This is significant as it reflects on the central support from the hips. This gives us a sense of balance and connectedness; it makes us stand and walk with easier strides.

Why this emphasis on the hip joint width distance? Think of the weight-bearing path of the body as an inverted Y. The weight of the body which is carried down through the spine gets divided at the end of the spine. It gets transferred to the hip joints on each side, passes through the centre of the knee joints and ends at the ankles. Feet, at hip joint width, permit the weight to be transmitted through this axis. If the feet are kept wider, the weight transmission is disturbed and the knees and the ankles suffer.

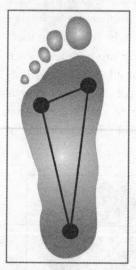

Weight-bearing points

Standing on All Threes: Don't worry! You do not have to go on your knees and palms to take care of your feet. All you need to do is spread your body's weight evenly on the three weight-bearing parts of your feet – the two sets of toe mounds (the first and the fifth toes) and the heels. Feel your weight equally between:

- both your feet
- the front and the back of each foot and
- the two sides of each foot.

The feet function best and provide the healthiest foundation when the arches are strong and the 'three corners' of each foot are in balance. The 'three corners' being:

- the mound of the big toe
- the mound of the little toe
- the center of the heel.

These 'Stand Smart' techniques bring about a straight and thus elegant stance too.

Do It Right – Walk Well

On an average, we take about 10,000 steps in a day. As we transfer the movement from one leg to the other, the body's weight gets distributed. So, we need to adjust and shift our balance sideways for a fine walk. When all these movements occur simultaneously, in co-ordination, we make the most efficient use of the joints and the soft tissues to create fluidity and ease of movement.

- The heel is our very first point of contact with the ground. It acts as a compass as well.

- The middle part of the foot is resilient and adapts to varied degrees of pressure when we walk. The pressure actually moves from muscle to muscle while this part works as a shock absorber and a pressure gauge.

- The toe mounds and the toes should be used to move forward when we push off from the toes. This is how the body should move forward.

Do It Right – Arch Fixes

Here are a few quick exercises to help correct wrong foot alignments. These exercises also help build the muscles that hold the feet's arches up; so, they are a slow but sure way of developing arches. Of course, a flat foot will not magically develop an arch, but it can become better than what it is.

For best results, do each exercise twice a day. Worry not; all the exercises together should not take more than five minutes. Also, whether they require you to sit or stand, do so in a comfortable, stable position. Place your feet well on the floor, that is:

- Spread your weight evenly on both your feet.
- Within each foot, spread the weight evenly between the two edges, the toe mounds and the heels.

Toe Fan

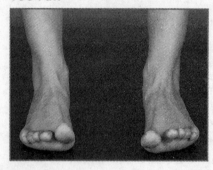

- You can stand or sit for the 'toe fan'.
- Press the mounds of your toes on th   e floor.
- Raise your toes off the floor.
- Fan them out and hold for ten seconds.
- Release your toes.
- Repeat ten times.

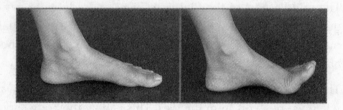

Flat foot (left); Arch with toe fan (right)

Toe Curls

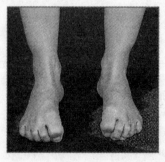

- You can stand or sit for the 'toe curls'.
- Curl your toes in as if you were asked to pick up tiny pieces of paper from the floor.
- Release your toes and curl them in again.
- Repeat for a minute.

Toe Walk

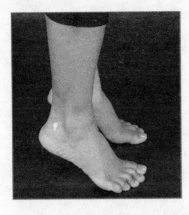

- Stand on the mounds of your toes.
- Walk on the mounds.
- Continue for a minute.

Outer-Edge Walk

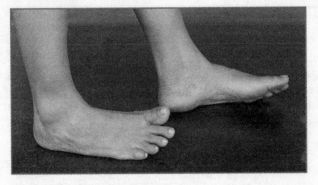

- Stand on the outer edges of both your feet. The little toes will touch the floor, right up to the heels' outer edges.
- Walk on the outer edges of your feet.
- Continue for a minute.

Calf Stretch: As you sit comfortably, lift one leg straight up at the knee. The other leg rests on the floor.
- Turn the toes of the lifted foot towards yourself. Push the ankle away.
- Feel the lovely stretch at the back of your lower leg (calf muscle).

- Hold for a minute.
- Repeat with the other leg.

Hip Clench

Please Refer to page 48, Chapter 6.
Notice the effect of a tone at the hips on your feet's arches:
- The mound of the big toe presses on the floor.
- Feel the arches of the feet lift up.
- Feel the stretch in the lower back.

Do It Right – Good Footwear

Comfortable standing or walking is first and foremost related to good shoes. What kinds of shoes are good for you?

- Shoes should have flexible soles – both in length and width. This permits a natural roll from the heels to the mounds of the toes while walking.

- Closed shoes should be slightly longer, broad toed and flat. You should be able to stretch and wriggle the toes inside so that they can be straight.

- Be careful while picking shoes that have a built-in arch. They work well only if they lift the foot correctly. It is best to use shoes with customized insoles for flat feet.

- Early footwear for children: Shoes play a vital role in the growth of a child's feet. When a child starts wearing footwear it is very important. If a child is made to start wearing shoes at a very young age and for long stretches of time, the natural development of functional arches gets warped. So, it is recommended to wait until the gait pattern of the child has firmly stabilized. Encourage children to play barefoot at home, in the garden or on the beach. In fact, as a parent, you can join in too and have fun.

Chain Reaction

Walking requires synchronization between multiple body parts – arms, spine, pelvis, hips, knees and feet. If the walk is devoid of smartness, certain muscles are underused, while others are overused. Either way, the muscles become vulnerable to injury and degeneration. Every step taken becomes a direct assault not just on the feet, but also on the hips and the knees, causing them to suffer wear and tear.

Similarly, stiff hips or knees have a crippling effect on the feet, as they make it difficult for the feet to establish proper contact with the ground while walking or even standing. This triggers an undesirable chain reaction in the body, which manifests in the form of gripped toes, anguished breathing, tight jaw-line and facial contortions. The existing discomfort becomes worse and there is further compression of the joints and reduction in the mobility.

Even faulty feet placement while standing affects the whole body. As the weight is improperly placed on the feet, the natural arches get distorted and the knees tend to lock. We try to adjust to this by thrusting our hips forward, which however sways the lower back in an excessively forward position. This can pressurize the muscles of the lower back, as they adapt themselves to shorter lengths, and hamper the blood supply to the lower back and the legs in general.

Each and every part of the body supports and affects the adjacent parts. Having discussed feet, where posture begins, we move up along the body axis to the knees.

Chapter 9

THE WEIGHT BEARERS – OUR KNEES

True alignment means that the inner mind reaches
every cell and fibre of the body.
~ BKS Iyengar

I had never imagined knee pain could be such a common issue. It is not only the middle aged and the elderly who come complaining about it; knee pain is surprisingly prevalent even among teenagers and young adults. I have finally given up counting the various types of knee problems – osteoarthritis, patellofemoral syndrome, bursitis, chondromalacia, locked knees. What I know is this – all these maladies are directly related to the condition that the knees are subjected to. The condition may occur either due to problems in other weight-bearing joints or due to the functional health of the muscles that support the knees.

Structure

The knee joint is a very fragile structure with a disposition to pain, disability and restricted movement, more than any other joint in the body. It would be valuable to understand its basic structure and mechanism.

The knee joint is formed at the lower end of the thigh bone and the upper ends of the two lower leg bones. The kneecap or the patella is a small, oval-shaped bone, which is embedded in the muscles that cover the knee. It is designed to protect the knee, increase smooth movement and reduce friction. When the leg moves, the kneecap glides up and down in a groove at the lower end of the thigh bone. It ideally remains centred or 'tracked' in its groove as the leg bends or straightens.

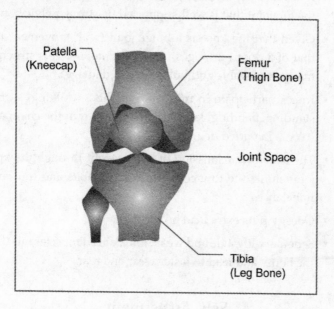

Structure of the knee joint

The suppleness, the strength and the balance of the muscles around the knees automatically reduces the friction in the joint. This keeps the knees in a healthy condition. The stronger the supporting muscles, the better the stability of the frame.

Front Thigh Muscles or the Quadriceps: Better known as 'quads', their contraction straightens the leg at the knee. The quadriceps group is made of four muscles, which meet at the knee joint. The kneecap is wrapped inside the lower end of the quadriceps muscles.

Back Thigh muscles or the Hamstrings: Hamstrings are a group of muscles that start behind the hips and run through to the back of the knees. Together they contract to bend the leg at the knee.

Other important things to understand the knee joint better are:

- It supports the entire body's weight.

- It has no bony structures to support it unlike, for example, the hip joint that is well-supported by strong pelvic bones.

- Given that the knee is a hinge joint (with movement like that of a door on hinges), it is very mobile. This structure makes it unstable and vulnerable to damage.

- Knees participate in most movements – walking, sitting, standing, bending, kneeling, rising up from the chair, and so on – in varied degrees.

- The axis of transmission of bodyweight through the knee joint shifts due to incorrect postural habits and muscular imbalances.

- Obesity puts extra load on the joint.

- Sedentary lifestyle and weak, imbalanced muscles misalign the bones and lead to faster wear and tear.

Self-Assessment

Ask someone to mark a dot at the centre of each of your kneecaps. Have them make another set at the end of your lower leg (shin) in the front. This would be exactly where the foot starts. Ideally, the line that joins the dots on each leg is vertical and perpendicular to the ground. In case the knees are dysfunctional, they are either inside or outside of this vertical line. The other questions you need to answer are:

- Where do the knees point – forward, or are they turned in or out?

- Are both knees at the same level in relation to each other?

- Are the knees hyper-extended, that is, pushed behind (locked)?

- Track your knees as you bend them simultaneously. Do they face the front, converge towards each other (knock knees) or diverge from each other (bowed legs) with the bend?

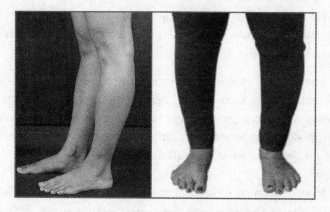

Knee alignment – locked knees and bow legs

Seen from the side, the knees should be in an easy, neutral position – neither too bent nor pushed behind in a locked position. The back of the knees should feel soft unlike the discomfort experienced when standing with absolutely stretched-out knees.

Seen from the front, the kneecaps are a guide to the alignment of the knees. They should point in the front, straight ahead. The knees should be in line with the second toe of the respective feet. If the knees get angled, inward or outward, or if they come together on bending, or separate widely when straightened, then there is an imbalance in the muscles that bend and straighten the knees.

Depending on the assessment of your knees, you will find a solution/correction in the next chapter.

Common Observations

Women are more susceptible to an early onset of age-related knee pain in comparison to men.

- **Mechanics:** The wider dimensions of the hip (pelvic) region in a woman's body increase the angle at the hip joint. This predisposes the knee joint to greater stress.

- **Hormones:** Strong muscles act as a protective mechanism for the joints. However, women lack androgen hormones, which help in the development of powerful muscles. Also, in the post-menopausal phase of life, the vital oestrogen hormone reduces, leading to further loss of muscle mass and tone.

Men too are prone to knee pain, but the reasons tend to be different. Due to their natural hormonal composition, men are blessed with stronger muscles. However, the downside is that their muscles are prone to become tight and short with overuse. Thus, it becomes more difficult for men to straighten their tight knees.

Men or women follow set patterns and lifestyles that affect their knee joints. However, because the causes are different, different solutions are in order.

Locked knees: Over-straightened and pushed back knees are known as locked knees. Knees are locked when we stand with all our weight on the heels. This happens due to the muscles behind the knees being weak, which makes the weight shift to the bones instead of to the muscles. The kneecaps push behind to smash into the joint space.

Other consequences of locked knees:

- Locked knees weaken the quads by making them lose tone and become loose. As the quads lose strength, they become flabby and soft. This sags the kneecap further into misalignment.

- Major nerves and veins pass from behind the knee. These get compressed when the knees are locked, leading to chronic leg pain, trouble with varicose veins, and other problems.

- Locked knees do not engage abdominal muscles, causing them to weaken. This then makes the lower back sway behind and form an unhealthy arch. Needless to say, the weight-bearing axis gets disturbed.

Incorrect Standing Habits: As mentioned in the previous chapter, the chain reaction to incorrect standing habits passes through the knees. When the feet are placed like a V, both the knees get pushed back in the locked position. This shifts the weight-bearing axis inward – from the centre of the knee joint towards the midline of the body – making the inner side of the knee joint bear more weight. This is why pain is felt on the inner side of the affected knee.

Patellofemoral Syndrome: Often misunderstood as knee arthritis, this is a very common and an easily manageable cause of knee pain. Here, the kneecap gets pulled horizontally to one side. Usually, there is an imbalance between the inner and the outer thigh muscles that form part of the quads group. In the tug-of-war between the two, the kneecap gets pulled to the side of the comparatively stronger muscle. This causes gritting and friction with the ends of the thigh bone, and results in inflammation and pain. Activities like walking, bending knees, using stairs, squatting or bending down hurt. What seems to be a case of arthritis is in all probability a case of patella maltracking. The answer to the problem lies in strengthening the quadriceps in a balanced way.

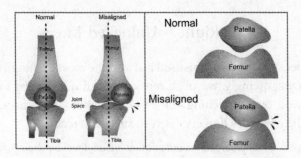

Patellofemoral syndrome:
misalignment of the kneecap (patella) in relation to the thigh bone (femur)

Sitting in a Chair for Long Hours: Our 'chaired' and sedentary lifestyle encourages tightened and shortened hamstrings as they remain contracted to keep the knees bent. The front thigh muscles, or the quads, get weakened since they are not used at all. This imbalance created between the short hamstrings and the under-toned quadriceps gets worse with time and impacts the knees.

Sitting with Crossed Legs: As mentioned earlier, crossing one knee over the other while sitting on a chair is fashionable and makes a style statement, but it eventually causes great damage to the knees. This position of the legs damages the lower knee, which tightens under the weight of the leg placed over it. The knee which crosses over also gets affected but in a different way.

You can try this for yourself. Sit with your right leg crossed over the left. Notice the right foot. It rotates and turns outward. Sitting in this position puts a strain on the ligaments inside the knee joint and, if done for long hours, creates an imbalance between the muscles that rotate the knee joint. The left knee too can suffer due to the constant inward pull on the left thigh with the weight of the right thigh on it.

The chair – perhaps the most commonly used furniture – has inadvertently brought in a host of postural maladies. It may be wise to introduce a daily practice of squatting on the floor.

Do It Right – Unlocked Knees

The knees are the most misused but also the most easily corrected joint. Unknowingly, we push our knees behind, thereby locking them and over-stretching the muscles behind the knees. This unhealthy practice however is very simple to rectify.

- Spread your weight evenly over your feet by bringing the weight of your body slightly to the front part of your feet.

- The knees will feel soft and relaxed rather than taut and tense.

Do It Right – Bring Back Lost Tone

As we know now, a joint is not an independent entity. We have to strengthen the muscles that hold the said joint in place. It is just a matter of bringing in a gentle tone to the muscles that support the knee by doing the following:

Hip Clench – Refer to page 48, Chapter 6.

This practice:

- Tones the weak thigh muscles at the front (quads).
- Makes the sagging kneecap pull up automatically.

Cartilage damage, softened kneecap, damaged ligaments, cysts, and more problems can all be treated with medicines and surgical interventions, provided that the root cause is identified and treated. However, the secret to healthy knees is to develop strong yet supple, supporting muscles around the knees that will keep the knees aligned with the other weight-bearing joints. From years of experience, I have found the answer in yoga.

Chapter 10

CAPPING KNEE PROBLEMS

Any malady in your physical body was a lot longer in coming than it takes to release it.
~ Abraham Hicks

Yoga is a remarkable system, especially for increased strength and flexibility of knees, and as a protection against future injuries or problems. Doctors are now convinced of the effectiveness of yoga practices to treat patients who need rehabilitation from arthritis and even ligament injuries.

Benefits of Yoga

Contrary to common belief, yoga is not only about stretching tight muscles to increase flexibility; it is as much about making the muscles around each joint strong enough to keep the joints appropriately aligned.

Strengthens All the Muscles Involved: Knee problems are often related to mechanical issues with the kneecap, which also impact the ligaments. The high point of yoga therapy is that it helps strengthen both the inner and the outer quadriceps and therefore helps keep the kneecap in alignment. Physiotherapy typically focuses on strengthening the muscles that surround the knee to help support it, but fails to work on the development of all the muscles involved, the inner and the outer thigh muscles as well as the upper and the lower muscles. Yoga does it with class. It strengthens the quadriceps, the hamstrings, the calves and the ankles, all fairly consistently.

Brings Nutrition to the Joints: Yoga helps increase the blood flow to the joints, which in turn nourishes the surrounding ligaments. Most yoga poses require alternate squeezing and releasing of the muscles. This sends nutrient-rich blood to the area that is worked and aids in its healing.

Safety First – Protect Your Knees When You Practice Yoga

There are specific yoga postures that act as a great boon to the knees. Yet, there is no escape from being careful and knowing your limitations. If done incorrectly, a posture can injure the knees or worsen existing injuries, which is why it is important to listen carefully to the body. In case there is a tug in the knee or on its sides in any posture, it is best to discontinue the practice.

- **Focus on the placement of the feet**: Good body alignment begins with the correct position of the feet. Else, the knees tend to be the first joint to be affected by over-compensation. Make sure to push down through the three corners (as discussed on page 66, chapter 8) to distribute the body weight equally.

- **Make sure the knees are aligned over the ankles**: The knees should point towards the second toe of the respective feet. They should not fall in or out of this line in any asana that requires bent knees or lunges.

- **Be cautious when you straighten the knees**: It is easy to hyperextend (overstretch) knees, when the body, especially the hip joints, are tight. It seems easier to get deeper into postures through locked knees, but it must be avoided at all costs. It is important to distinguish between pulling the kneecaps up (okay to do) and locking the knees (not okay). If you have a tendency to hyperextend the knees, you should keep the knees slightly bent in the standing and the forward-folding poses.

Therapeutic Practices for the Knees

Knee problems can be dealt with the help of a number of therapeutic practices, which not only work on the knees but also help:

- Strengthen the arches of the feet.

- Distribute the body weight on the three corners of both the soles.

- Stretch the short and tight hamstrings (muscles behind the knee joint).

- Strengthen the weak quads (front thigh muscles).

- Balance the uneven contraction of quads by strengthening the inner thigh muscles.

Practices

Tadasana (Palm Tree Pose)

Activates feet

Standing in Tadasana is the best way to restore the natural strength and adaptability of the feet. In Tadasana, the essential structure of the foot can be represented by a triangle formed between three points on the sole – the middle of the heel, the mound of the great toe and the mound of the fifth toe. The imaginary lines that connect these points represent the arches, the three lines through which postural support is derived. It is easier to understand the mechanics of the foot with the assistance of a wall.

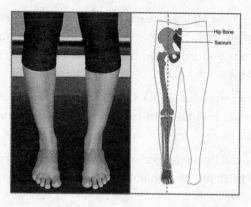

Standing in line with the weight-bearing axis

i.   Footprints on the Wall: Tadasana Alignments in the Lying down Position

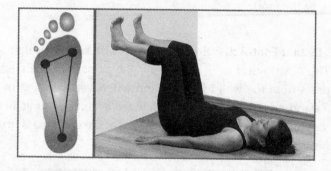

Triangle representing structure of the foot in tadasana

- The first step is to create footprints on the wall. The idea is to understand the exact mechanics of using the three points so that it can be applied when we stand and walk.

- Lie down on the floor on a mat, with the sole of your feet placed against a wall. The heels are just above the level of the knees and the thighs are perpendicular to the floor. Take a few smooth breaths to relax the body.

- Spread the toes and then gently press the mound under each toe into the wall.

- Now, press all ten toes equally. As they seem to imprint on the wall, stretch them out to lengthen them further. This practice will bring the balls of the feet into firm contact with the wall.

- As you maintain contact with the wall, lift all the toes off the wall. Feel the firm pressure of the toe mounds on the wall.

- Also, feel the wide area on which each heel can press firmly as if there are two points of deep contact on two edges of each heel.

- To complete the practice, stand up and absorb the same feeling by pressing the mounds of the toes and heels on the floor. The weight will be evenly distributed over the entire surface of the sole (and not just the heels or just one edge of the foot).

ii.   **Instant Foot-Activation Technique: Lift Your Toes up**
The next logical step is to apply the principles of the sole-press from the wall to the ground whenever we stand or do a standing yoga pose. Consolidate the action by lifting all ten toes off the floor. Notice how the base of the great toe is firmly pressed.

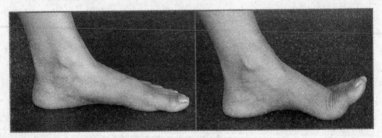

    This technique instantly activates the feet as the three weight-bearing points get grounded, the arches get naturally lifted, the heels press down, the base of the shin or the leg bone moves back and the inner leg gets engaged. The impossible, may we say, is so easily achieved.

People with flat feet can learn to develop a healthy arch by lifting the toes with more weight on the outer edge of the foot and the outer part of the heel. The technique is equally handy for people with knocked or bowed legs.

The above practice is a postural correction. The practices that follow are for those who experience knee pain. These are all muscle strengthening exercises which help bring the knee joint back in alignment.

For all practices that require you to sit, please use a firm chair.

- Make sure the height of the chair is such that your upper legs make a right angle with your lower legs.

- Your feet should be firm on the floor and should not hang from the chair. If your feet hang, slide forward on the chair until the feet are firmly placed on the floor.

- Keep your legs parallel and at hip-width distance from each other.

Aided Utkatasana Variation (Chair Pose)

Activates and aligns quadriceps

Opposite action on muscles serves to stabilize and align the knees safely in all positions and during all kinds of movements. Utkatasana, or the chair pose, strengthens the knee joints and the weak inner leg muscles, and aligns the feet, the ankles and the hips with the knees. Once the principle of this revolutionary asana is understood, the practice can be innovatively integrated into daily activities.

i.   **Hand Press Technique:**

- Sit on a firm chair.
- Lean forward from the hips and place the hands on the outside of the legs, just below the knees. Alternatively, press

a folded cushion or blanket between the knees instead of using the hands.

- Make the thigh muscles firm. While the hands strongly push in towards the midline, press your thighs out with an equal force.

- Hold for ten counts. Do not hold your breath.

- This restricted isometric practice will not only align the legs but will also release the compression in the hips. The technique can be used to advantage even when we stand.

- Release the hand-press and relax your muscles.

- Repeat ten times.

ii.   Knee Alignment with Belt:

- Sit on a firm chair.

- Tie a cloth or a belt around the legs just below the knees.

- Try to separate the thighs against the resistance of the belt, such that your thighs try to open the belt while the belt does not give in to the pressure. Feel the impact. So, your thighs try to open the belt while the belt doesn't give up.

- Hold for ten counts. Keep breathing.

- Release the resistance of the belt and relax the muscles.

- Repeat ten times.

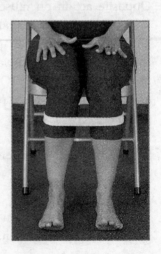

This simple practice can relieve knee pain, which is sometimes wrongly attributed to knee arthritis. The real cause of the pain is maltracked kneecap or the patellofemoral syndrome. However, if it is not managed at an early stage it *can* lead to arthritis.

Bolster Lift

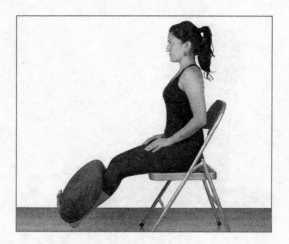

Strengthens outer thigh muscles

- Sit on a firm chair. Slide your hips a little towards the outer edge of the chair.

- Place a bolster at your ankles. You will need to turn your feet up at your ankles to hold the bolster in position. Please do not use weights on each leg individually because this would beat the purpose of this practice. This practice is designed such that you use both legs in tandem.

- Once you have balanced the bolster on your ankles, lift the bolster up till knee level.

- Make sure you do not let your upper body lean backward. Keep your hands on the chair beside your hips to avoid the lean.

- Hold the legs in the raised leg position for ten counts. Make sure you are breathing.

- Bring your legs down only half way.

- Gently raise them up to knee level again to hold for another ten counts.

- Repeat eight to ten times.

Dandasana (Staff Pose)

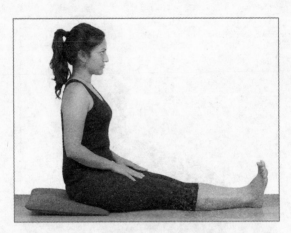

Activates quadriceps and lengthens hamstrings

- Sit on the floor on a mat or sit on a firm bed. Stretch your legs out.
- Keep your feet together.
- Point your toes up towards the ceiling.
- If you have a stiff back or feel a strain on the back, place a folded blanket or a cushion under your hips. This will keep the pelvis free and help lengthen the back with ease.
- Squeeze your thighs. Make your thigh muscles hug your thigh bone. This pulls your kneecap up towards your torso and ensures that you do not hyperextend your knees.
- If at first it is too strenuous to make your legs straight, you can put a rolled blanket under your knees to give you support. Over time, as your hamstrings start stretching, you can reduce the support. Also, if the heels leave the floor, they can overextend the knees. In this case too, place a rolled towel under the knees to prevent hyperextension.
- The trunk should maintain a right angle to the legs, with the top of the head directly over the tail bone region.
- Keep your palms on the floor next to the hips. Do not sink

on the arms. Instead, try to gently lift them, lengthening the back from the tail bone to the neck and head.

- Lower your shoulders. Maintain a slight bend at the elbows to relax the shoulders.

- Get ready for a quadriceps work out. The front thigh muscles will contract and give a little upward pull to the kneecaps. This action should not push the thighs and the shin bones down towards the floor but should draw the kneecaps gently towards the hips.

- Very weak, flabby and unused quadriceps will not respond immediately but will definitely do so with repeated practice.

- Once you are familiar with the working of the quads in the staff pose, maintain the pose for a longer time. Try to lengthen the legs from the hips to the heels and firm the quads just above the inner knees.

- Hold the pose for about a minute. Breathe easily and steadily, and do not let your heels leave the ground.

- Having learnt the technique of using the quads without hyperextending the knees, you can now safely apply it while standing or performing other activities that use the knee joint.

Regular practice of the staff pose helps the knees tremendously. So powerful is this asana that it can bring about a normal alignment from the toes to the head.

Single Leg Raises

Strengthen quadriceps and hamstrings

- Lie down on the floor with folded legs.
- Imprint your back. (ref to page 115, Chapter 12.)
- Straighten the right leg out.
- Squeeze the thigh and the hips gently.

- Turn the toes in to point towards you, stretching the back of the leg.
- Lift the leg up till the right thigh is at the same level as the left.
- Hold for ten counts as you continue to breathe.
- Bring the leg down without letting the heel touch the ground.
- Repeat five times.
- Point the toes out to stretch the front of the leg.
- Repeat with the other leg.

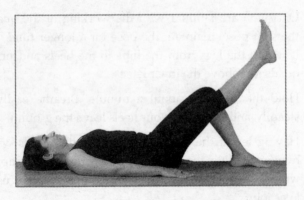

Side Leg Raises

Strengthen outer thighs

- Lie down on your side with your legs stretched out straight. If you have a sensitive lower back, you can fold the lower leg.
- Make sure your upper shoulder and upper hip are on top of the lower shoulder and lower hip, that is, you are not leaning forward or behind at the shoulder or the hip.
- Tuck your navel in.
- Squeeze the upper thigh and the hips gently.

- Turn the toes in to point towards you, stretching the back of the leg.

- Lift the leg up by a few inches (not all the way up).

- Hold for ten counts as you continue to breathe.

- Bring the leg down without letting the heel rest completely.

- Repeat five times.

- Point the toes out to stretch the front of the leg.

- Turn on to the other side; repeat with the other leg.

Supta Padangusthasana with Belt
(Supine Hand-to-Toe Pose)

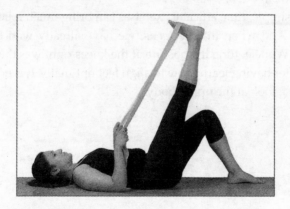

Stretches tight hamstrings, with a relaxed back

- Lie down on the floor with folded legs.
- Imprint your back. (Refer to page 115, Chapter 12.)
- Wrap a band / belt / cotton stole around the left sole.
- Bend your elbows and pull the thigh towards you.
- Do not allow the hips to lift off the ground and let the right foot remain folded, with the foot firm on the mat. Take a couple of deep breaths.

- This assures a hamstring stretch within safe range.
- With the left leg vertical, activate the quadriceps by pulling the kneecap.
- Try to lengthen the leg by pushing the left heel away from you.
- Breathe smoothly and naturally. Hold for a minute.
- To come out of the pose, bring down the left leg gradually and gracefully.
- Repeat with the other leg.

Reverse Walking

Refer to page 158, Chapter 17
These simple, time efficient exercises can bring much relief to the knees. And when that happens, we have already won half the battle. While getting the posture at the knees right was the logical step after having learnt how to align feet optimally. It is now time to take a look at the upper body.

Chapter 11

OUR BEAM – THE S SPINE

You must learn to be still in the midst of activity and
to be vibrantly alive in repose.
~ Indira Gandhi

Thanks to the spine, our body works as an anti-gravity machine. The spine is a shaft – a strong bony structure made of 33 interlocking bony segments called vertebrae. These are stacked one on top of the other. The spine is designed to be flexible and supple. It protects within its cage the 'life cable' – the vital spinal cord.

The spinal cord is accorded this importance because it is an extension of the brain. It has minuscule nerves coming out through the space between the vertebrae. These nerves extend out to the rest of the body. The spine and the spinal cord coordinate all the neuromuscular activities that connect the brain with the minutest parts of the body.

Structure

A basic understanding of the spine structure will help us know the reasons and solutions for the very common backaches.

Special S curve: The spine has three slight curves along its length and makes a gentle S curve from the neck to the tailbone. This shape gives flexibility and resilience to the back. The spine behaves like a shock absorber, provides stability and facilitates smooth movement of the back. When the curves of the spine match the natural specifications, the vertebrae are stacked precisely one on top of the other. When the curvature increases or decreases, joints lose their precision, and the adjoining bones put unwanted pressure on one another, causing grinding pain.

The vertebrae of the spine are divided into four regions. Their structure and nomenclature is based on their location.

- Cervical: At the level of the neck and the shoulder (C1 to C7, refer to the image given below).

- Thoracic: Behind the chest, through the upper and middle back or the torso (T1 to T12, Figure refer to the image given below).

- Lumbar: Behind the abdominal organs, at the level of the lower back (L1 to L5, refer to the image given below).

- Sacral: Continuing further down the spine, lower on the back, just above our hips, to form the tailbone (refer to the image given below).

The cervical and the lumbar regions have a mild concavity – a mild C shape with the bump towards the front of the body. The thoracic region has a mild convexity – a mild C shape with the bump away from the body. This together makes for the S shape of the spine.

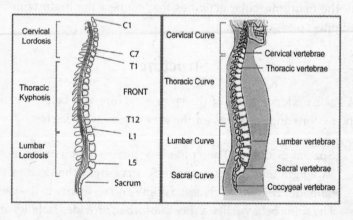

Vertebrae of the spine and regions of the spine

Discs: Between each pair of vertebrae are circular pads or cushion-like structures called discs. These are natural protective cushions that help with weight transmission. They also act as shock absorbers during various movements. At birth, 80% of each disc is made of water. In a healthy spine, the discs are plump and thick. Discs tend to become dry with prolonged sitting, low water intake, lack of exercise and, of course, aging.

Pelvis: This is a bony basin that forms the lower part of the trunk. It connects the base of the spine to the lower limbs. In human beings, the pelvis is unique because it offers tremendous strength and flexibility to the back. This girdle like structure, which supports the spine and the hip joints, is the fulcrum of our upright posture. It works as a junction to align the upper and lower parts of the body, thus acting as a central balancing mechanism.

Muscles

i.   **Paraspinal Muscles behind the Spine:** These are a group of thick, strong muscles behind the spine. They start at the base of the skull and span over the entire length of the spine, down to the lower back. They connect each vertebra to the vertebra above and below it and finally wrap behind the pelvis, on which the spine is supported. These muscles are completely responsible for maintaining proper posture. You have to remember to keep them well-toned; else the spine may become vulnerable and collapse.

ii. **Muscles Connecting the Upper Body to the Lower Body:** The psoas is a large muscle that originates at each side of the lower spine, goes through the abdominal cavity at the hip and reaches each thigh. The psoas muscles allow us to raise the thighs towards the upper body. If they are tight, they can pull the lower back into an arch.

iii. **Abdominal Muscles in Front:** Layers and fibres of muscles criss-cross to support the organs in the abdominal region and the lower back. Strong abdominal muscles, popularly known as abs, play a dual role. They shape the front part of the trunk and also lend protective support to the spine. Abs are very important to stabilize the lower back as there is no other bony/hard support in the front part of the trunk. The strength of these muscles is crucial to the health of the spine.

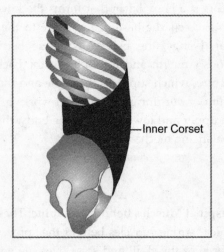

Abdominal support to the lower back

iv. **Muscles at the Hip**: The gluteal muscles or the gluts form the buttocks. They help keep the hip in line with the rest of the body. If they are weak, they allow the pelvis to tilt forward, increasing the lower back arch. Prolonged activities, like sitting for long hours on a chair, weaken these muscles.

B. Self-Assessment

It will be nice to know some simple techniques of assessing the back. They are:

Lower Back Curvature

- Stand barefoot with your back to the wall. Keep your heels one to two inches away from the wall, so that the hips lightly brush the wall.

- Insert a palm between the lower back and the wall. Observe the gap.

- Ideally, there should be a slight arch, a concavity in the lower back – neither too much nor too little – allowing the palm to fit in the space.

Lower back curvature can be assessed as:

- Normal arch (Just enough space for the palm to pass between your back and the wall).

- Over arched or sway back (Lots of room left after inserting the palm).

  - Your belly protrudes out.

  - Your abdomen feels too lax or loose.

  - Your knees lock behind.

- Flat back (Difficult to insert the palm).

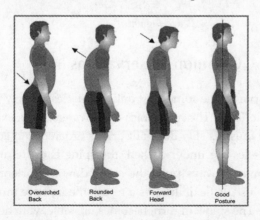

Lower back curvature

Pelvic Alignment

The pelvis is not a fixed structure; it is significantly mobile. Its mobility determines the health of the entire body, specifically that of the back. The pelvis has to be at a correct angle to function optimally. An aligned pelvis is anteverted in position, that is, it tilts forward slightly. This forward tilt accommodates the wedge of the lower spine perfectly. Any other position of the pelvis compromises the lower spine and pressurizes it. If your hips jut out or the lower belly pouches out, your pelvis is not in alignment.

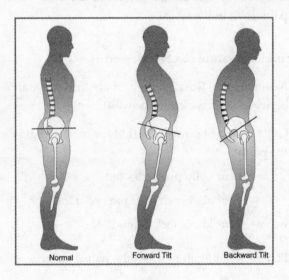

Pelvic alignment

Common Observations

The natural curves of the spine exist only if muscles actively work to keep them in form. The mechanics and arrangements exist. It is just that the muscles stay dormant unless ordered into action. When the muscles are underworked, the spine is at the mercy of gravity. Gravity always pulls the spine down, shortening it and making it lose its flexibility. As a result, the inactive muscles start to shrink. The spine, in turn, becomes unstable, with altered curvatures. This can lead to a lot of pain.

Arched Lower Back or Swayback: We all have a small curve in our lower back or the lumbar region. When this curve increases beyond a designated limit, it is called swayback or increased lordosis.

A healthy forward-tilt of the pelvis should be at the lumbosacral angle – the angle between the last vertebra at the lower back (lower lumbar region or L5) and the tail-bone region (sacrum or S1). This gives a natural curve placed very low in the spine.

Swayback (lordosis) is a deeper curvature of the lumbar spine. It is common to see people with an overarched lower back. Swayback is associated with the following:

- The belly is lax because of weak abdominal muscles.

- It sags forward to protrude beyond the line of the belt.

- It pulls the abdominal organs and the lower back forward.

- The spine slackens with the forward tension.

- To compensate, the muscles behind the spine contract and eventually tighten.

- The buttocks stick back, further accentuating the arch.

- The imbalance between the abdominal and spinal muscles compresses the discs in the lower back, which leads to pain.

With this, the weight of the body, which should have been evenly distributed over the entire lumbar curve, concentrates at the peak of the arch – at L3-L4 and L4-L5 disc spaces. This pressure at the centre of the arch allows abnormal movements between the vertebrae, which lead to disc damage. If not corrected, the discs gyrate and shrink and the vertebrae grate against each other, eventually leading to spondylitis.

A swayback is commonly seen in women with a flabby and toneless abdomen, especially post-pregnancy. Obese men with a pot belly too have it due to weak abdominals. The good news is that exercises that strengthen abdominal muscles and stretch the tight back muscles reduce this excessive curvature and reverse the compression of the discs.

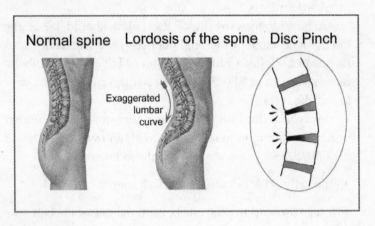

Normal spine (natural curve), swayback or lordosis (exaggerated curve) and disc pinch

Pain associated with an arched back usually follows the following pattern:

- Body type: usually short, overweight, large abdomen and with a large buttock or hip area.

- Lifestyle: those who spend a lot of their time seated with a stretched out lumbar spine or are in professions that involve reaching out like while horse riding, driving a two wheeler, etc.

- The pain worsens on standing and improves on sitting.

- The pain reduces when the legs are bent at the hips and brought up.

- When returning from a forward bend, the pain precipitates with the straightening of the back. This pain can be prevented by coming up correctly from the bent position. (Refer to page 198, Chapter 22.)

- It is difficult to flatten the lower back when lying down, as the pain worsens on lying down on the back, especially with straight legs.

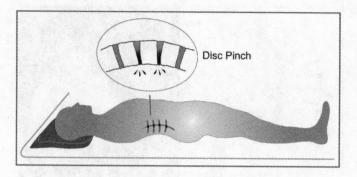

Disc pinch experienced by people with an arched back

Flat and Rounded Lower Back: A flat or rounded lower back results in the pelvis being tilted back. The natural curvature of the lower back becomes less than normal. The lower back is almost flat due to weak muscles, which are unable to hold the body up. In such cases, the hips (gluteal muscles) are small and flabby. When people with flat backs wear trousers, the trousers tend to slide down. Also, when a trouser belt is worn, it appears higher in the front than in the back.

Again, we see that:

- the loss of the normal curvature interferes with the shock absorption of the spine;

- supports of the spine become tight and the vertebrae compress;

- The lower back discs suffer from undue pressure and tend to bulge out of the spine.

This can be seen in exercise buffs who carve out the fashionable six pack abs. The workout builds extra tight abdominal muscles, the repercussions of which are unforeseen in the beginning. An abnormally tight abdomen pulls up the pelvis, flattens the lower back and obviously damages the postural alignment.

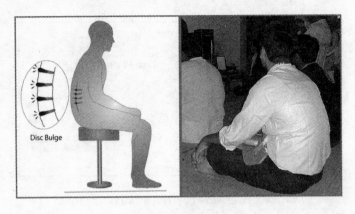

Sitting with rounded back

Sitting for long hours with a rounded back compresses the discs and squeezes the vital water content out from their centre. As a result of the loss of water, the fibrous rim of the discs gets dry and frizzy, and leads to tears and cracks. Sometimes a soft, pulpy cushion of a disc oozes out from the tears and the cracks. The disc then impinges on the nerves and the surrounding tissues, causing pain. This is commonly known as PID or Prolapsed Intervertebral Disc or herniated disc.

The joint space between the vertebrae may eventually reduce. Every small movement then creates friction and leads to wear and tear. A sudden increase in the intra-abdominal pressure, such as when you sneeze or bend suddenly, causes extensive damage. Postural corrections go a long way in preventing disc compression.

The pain associated with rounded backs has the following features:

- It generally affects people with a tall and slender build, usually males.

- Those who spend a lot of time seated, with the lower back rounded from behind, are also prone to it.

- The pain worsens on sitting and improves on standing.

- It increases on casual forward bending when the spine rounds itself. It can be prevented by bending the right way (hip hinged and knees bent – Refer to page 196, chapter 22).

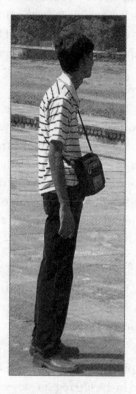

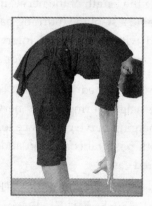

Disc Bulge

Wrong forward bending

Flat back

Tight Hip Muscles: The psoas muscles present in the front part of the hips are usually overused and tight due to the habit of being chair-bound. On lying down on the back with straight legs, the overtight psoas muscles push the lower spine forward. This strains the vertebrae at the lower back, often resulting in the pinched sciatic roots. This handicap can be overcome by adopting a simple procedure. (Refer to page 121, chapter 12.)

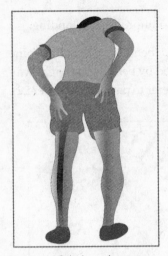

Sciatica pain

Sciatica: The shooting pain of sciatica is a dreaded one. It occurs due to compression of the sciatic nerve due to a number of reasons. The sciatic nerve originates at the lower back, emerges from the thigh and runs down the legs to meet the feet on the outer sides. This nerve may get pinched as a result of an altered spinal structure.

The space for the nerve to pass through narrows down with compression at the joint from where it originates. This leads to pain along the length of the nerve. It could vary from being a dull ache to being a stabbing, burning pain. Sciatica pain is commonly associated with a prolapsed intervertebral disc. There are two more common postural reasons for sciatica pain.

- An overarched lower back could compress the discs and the neighbouring sciatic nerve, giving rise to pain. If the emerging nerve gets space to exist, the pain can disappear. With postural correction and simple exercises, this can be cured easily.

- The Piriformis Syndrome – The piriformis is a deep muscle, which can be felt like a tight band in the hip region, when we sit cross-legged on the floor. The sciatic nerve is placed just under it. Piriformis syndrome occurs when pressure is applied on the sciatic nerve by the tight piriformis muscle.

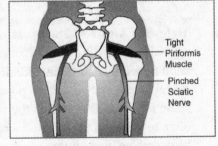

Tight
Piriformis
Muscle

Pinched
Sciatic
Nerve

Piriformis syndrome
(postural cause of sciatica)

Improper sitting habits and lack of squatting result in tight piriformis muscle. Some simple stretches can help manage pain. A complete recovery from this nagging handicap is also possible.

If in pain, study it.

A chronic pain in the back cannot be 'fixed' until we study and understand the underlying reasons. The reason could be any of the ones discussed so far – a swayback, a rounded back and so on. Fortunately, most of these causes can be traced to our own habitual movement patterns, so the 'fix' is in our control too.

Sometimes even the best of professionals need guidance on actively taking control of their health. Those programmed with better body awareness are able to recover fast. Body awareness does not imply bookish knowledge or information downloaded from the Internet (half knowledge can be dangerous). It is a mindful journey of learning to value the body and its creator.

Acute backache does not happen overnight and does not disappear overnight. It is necessary to have faith, be open-minded and positive; after all, attitude matters in all walks of life! In order to get long-term relief from back pain, we have to:

- identify the postural habits that could have led to muscle imbalances.

- work towards healing muscles with an appropriate mix of stretches and muscle strengthening exercises.

- apply corrective principles in our day-to-day activities.

Do It Right – Engage Your Belly

We need a strong inner belt to keep us away from the elastic lumbar belts that people with disabling lower backache are required to wear. These external belts do not provide long-lasting support to the spine as the underlying muscles go lax, as if on a vacation. In fact, the muscles become weaker with prolonged use of these elastic belts. Loss of baseline tone of the TA muscles is a major cause of lower back aches and other problems like poor digestion and disordered ovarian function.

At this point, we should remind ourselves of the 'Breathe Out, Belly In; Breathe In, Belly Out' mantra. (Refer to page 49, Chapter 6.)

Do It Right – Pelvic Tilt or Neutral Pelvis

This is a very important step in reducing the curve of the lower back, improving the posture and getting rid of lower back discomforts. This is best understood lying down by imprinting the back as described in the next chapter on page 115, 119. When you lie down, gravity helps you tilt your pelvis and makes it easier to reduce the curve in the lower back. This comes in handy especially when you are in pain.

When you are not in pain:

- Stand with your back against the wall.
- Place your heels about six inches away from the wall.
- Keep your knees soft.
- Pull your belly button in.
- Gently push your lower back against the wall.
- Hold the posture for ten counts without holding the breath.
- Release and repeat a few times.

Over time you can do it without the wall by pulling the belly in towards the spine and letting the tailbone drop down slightly. Imagine you have a tail and a little child is pulling your imaginary tail down.

Another way to do the pelvic tilt:

- Observe your side profile in the mirror.
- Tip the belly region forward slightly. This will tilt your

pelvic basin towards the front and will increase the curvature of the lower back.

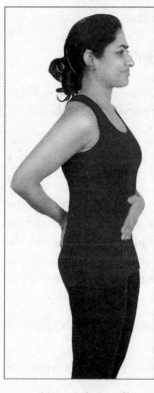

- If you overdo this, the belly will bulge out and you may feel a pressure on the lower back.

- Tilt the pelvis backward by squeezing the buttocks together and by tightening the muscles of the abdomen. This will tuck the tailbone in.

- Your back will flatten to provide adequate protection to the lower back.

Yet another way to do the pelvic tilt is as follows:

- Wear a belt just under the navel (NOT under the belly).

- At the front, slightly tilt the belt downward.

- Your pelvis will automatically tilt into alignment.

- Make sure you do not push your hips back to overdo the tilt.

Do It Right – Tone Your Hips

Hip clench – Refer to page 48, Chapter 6.
You can stand, sit or lie down to do this practice. In fact, you can do it as you walk too! See the effect of the hip clench on your lower back:

- It tones the core giving the lower back the much needed support.

- It helps bring the pelvis in the neutral position.

- It reduces the extra arch at the lower back.

Hold this gentle squeeze whenever you can.

A Fine-Tuned Spine

A healthy, well-supported spine is free from stress and tension as it engages smoothly in movements. For a fine-tuned spine:

- The vertebrae are stacked the way nature meant it, one over the other with comfortable space between them for the discs to fit.

- The natural S curvature of the spine is maintained. The spine should have a gentle, elongated curve and not an exaggerated S shape. It has a mild concavity behind the neck and the lower back (mild C shape, bump towards the front of the body) and a mild convexity behind the upper back region (mild C shape, bump away from the body).

- The pelvis is slightly tilted forward (at the lumbosacral or tailbone junction, not higher up).

- There is a baseline tone in the abdominal muscles to prevent an excessive forward pelvic tilt.

When the spine is not fine-tuned and the natural subtle curves of the spine get disturbed – reversed or exaggerated – the prognosis of a chronic backache is on the cards. Standing, sitting, driving, sleeping in the wrong manner, all worsen the condition. No wonder back pain has afflicted 90% of us at some or the other time in life. Let's empower ourselves to bring some relief.

Chapter 12

SPINE TUNING

Notice that the stiffest tree is most easily cracked, while the bamboo or willow survives by bending with the wind.
~ Bruce Lee

Back pain is like an unsolicited guest. It comes suddenly when all is well and gives a very grim turn to life. The early signs of discomfort tend to be conveniently ignored; signs telling you to 'Beware' or better still 'Be Aware'!

Be accountable to your body, respect it and work enthusiastically to keep all the muscles healthy and well-toned. Poor postural habits are the deep undercurrents of the body falling apart. Yet, we allow ourselves to get misled by myths.

Myths Related to Lower Backache

X-Rays Tell the Ultimate Cause of Back Pain: X-rays are important as they show the health of the bones and the joints. That said, x-rays, and for that matter even MRI scans, cannot detect the strength of and the balance between various muscles surrounding the bones. The state-of-the-art radiological equipment available today is still not capable of assessing muscle resilience.

As mentioned earlier, I have examined many people who suffer from backaches in spite of a clean chit from x-rays, just as I have examined those with gross wear and tear of bones revealed by x-rays, but who do not really suffer from pain. Wonder why? The problem and the solution lie inherently in the muscles. With healthy and functionally balanced muscles, you can stay free of pain despite a negative x-ray report.

Use of a Belt Helps and Supports the Back Forever: External corsets are prescribed for people with an unstable lower back. These are used to correct the distortion and to protect damaged tissues. Indiscriminate use of a lumbar belt actually creates more problems than it solves. The belt supports the spine, but when there is no acute problem, the back muscles stay unused and get shortened, resulting in stiffness and further degeneration.

Fitness Freaks Do Not Get Back Pain: Workouts can create muscle imbalances if we concentrate too heavily on certain areas of the body and neglect others. Runners, cyclists, bodybuilders can be candidates for back problems. Cyclists have serious muscle imbalances in the lower body and legs. Intensive use of the paddles overworks one set of muscles, while it underworks another. Body builders and fitness enthusiasts also fall prey to back pains.

Examine the story of Diniar, a successful 39-year old journalist, who epitomizes a life of health and fitness. He follows a strict workout regimen combined with excellent dietary habits. He thought he had an ace up his sleeve as far as robust health was concerned, until one day he was suddenly hospitalized for a bad back and promptly put on traction.

Diniar's colleague, Shekhar, who attended my yoga classes, narrated his plight. Diniar's exercise routine involved an hour-long daily swim followed by an hour of hectic gym and weight training. The pertinent question is where and why Diniar went wrong.

Diniar's is a classic case of imbalanced workout that involved only muscle strengthening while completely ignoring the equally important aspect of muscle stretching. In addition, he worked long hours in a slumped posture at the computer table. Moral of the story: not only do you need a correct balance between strengthening and stretching in your physical regimen, you must also back it by posture awareness 24 x 7.

'Surf Board Abs' Should Be the Aim: Today, the external look of the abdomen determines the level of fitness. While on one extreme, there are people who completely ignore their bodies, on the other there are those who pay too much attention to the way it looks from the outside. A protruding belly certainly causes backache. However, those with an extremely streamlined body, six-pack abs and broad shoulders also suffer from backache.

Men and women are getting obsessed with the physique displayed by film stars and models. Aping them is in vogue and though the short-term effect may be thrilling, it would be wise to be concerned about the long-term effect. Body-crafting specialists train the superficial abdominal muscles to remain in a contracted state. The look may be very appealing and worth applauding, but remember that in the process of achieving this look, these muscles get further tightened and shortened. This draws the chest and the pelvis close to each other, resulting in a flat lower back, which then puts extra pressure on the discs. The worst bit is that this restricts abdominal breathing and promotes unhealthy shallow chest breathing. The gait alters and soon becomes the root cause for failing health.

Common Errors While Practising Yoga

It is common to hear people complain of backache that began or increased after a couple of yoga sessions. Little do they realize that this is usually because of improper guidance or prescription of incorrect asanas. I have always believed that 'How We Do' matters more than 'What We Do' and this applies here more than anywhere else.

Forward bends with rounded backs: Instead of bending from the hips, many of us bend from the waist due to tight hamstrings (muscles at the back of the thighs). The aim of doing a forward bend is to stretch the back muscles, not to curve the spine. Forward bends should be done:

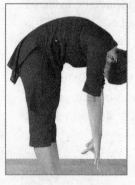

- with a straight lower back;
- with the abdomen pulled in;
- leading with the heart (not the head);
- from the hip joint.

Wrong – Forward bending with rounded lower back

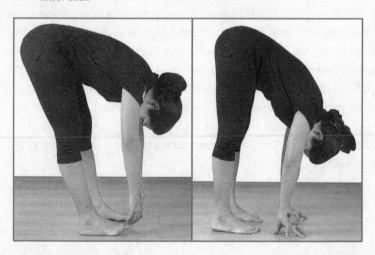

Wrong – Hips behind the ankles   *Right – hips in line with ankles*

Backward bends at the lower back: Backbends should not be an overarching of the lumbar spine. This is especially important for people with a swayback or increased lower back curvature as doing so compresses the bones and worsens the pressure on the discs. For example, Bhujangasana, or the Cobra Pose, is a backbend found in almost every yogic protocol. If done carelessly by people with an accentuated lumbar curvature, it can harm their lower back rather than offering any relief.

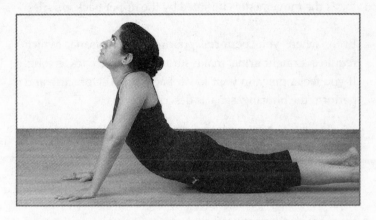

Wrong – Bhujangasana with over-arched back and sagging belly

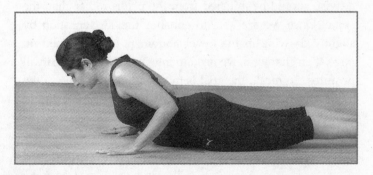

Right – Bhujangaasana with toned back and belly in

A backbend should be done with the following points in mind:

- Stabilize the lower spine and the tail area by gently bringing tone in the hips (gluteal muscles).

- Pull your navel in towards your spine.

- Lift the middle and the upper back away from the pelvis.

- Do not push up through the palms to extend and lift the back. Note that safe versions of backbends require bent elbows. Overuse of arms should be discouraged. Instead, the palms should be used for minimal support as the movement is initiated by the upper back muscles.

Even when you perform poorna bhujangasana, which requires straight arms, make sure your lower back is long. If you feel a pinch in your lower back, stop the practice and perform the bhujangasana as described above.

Asanas without involving the core: During yoga practices, the activity of the inner corset or the deep abdominal muscles is fundamental to the stabilization of the posture. This central support makes it possible to release the compensatory tension we carry in different parts of the body. A weak, sagging and toneless abdomen strains the back. Any yoga practice, even a twist, should be initiated from the pelvis rather than the spine. Once we are able to enhance the TA sensation by slightly drawing in the lower abdomen, as mentioned on page 47 in chapter 6, we need to integrate this practice in all postures. To recall, the goal is to sustain a mild tone in the inner corset during any activity and the contraction should be just 10-25% of the maximum.

Therapeutic Practices for the Back

The best things in life are simple ones. Here I share some simple core exercises that have to be done with awareness for quick and sustained results. They have no side effects; only positive results. Enjoy them.

Imprinted Lower Back

Tones abdominal muscles

This is a very effective technique to do away with the pain caused by excessive lower back curvature. It is like wearing a natural belt around the lower back, except that it is made up of your own muscles. It gives the lower back the much needed support.

- Lie down flat on your back. Bend your legs at the knees, your heels at a comfortable distance from the hips.

- As you exhale, pull the navel in and press your lower back towards the mat.

- This will slightly lift the tail bone away from the floor and cause the pelvis to roll back towards the floor. This engages all the belt muscles.

- Breathe with your chest as you hold the position for five to ten seconds.

- Inhale to relax.

- Repeat as many times as you can in the morning and before you sleep at night. You will be pleasantly surprised to see the pain disappear!

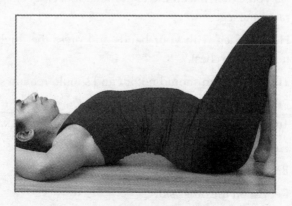

Wrong – Over-arched back

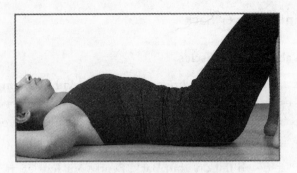

Right – Imprinted lower back to tone the core

This is one of the tools to understand the correct pelvic alignment mentioned on page 98, 106 in the previous chapter. The tilt in the pelvis observed in this practice should be applied when we stand or sit to keep it aligned.

Ardha-Pawanmuktasana (Half-Wind Release Pose or Half-Leg Lock Pose)

Stretches paraspinal muscles

- Lie down on your back with the legs bent.
- Imprint your back as explained in the previous practice.
- As you exhale, keep the abdominal muscles engaged and raise one leg.
- Hold the leg with your hands and press the thigh down towards the chest.
- The other thigh should not lift and should remain straight, pressed down.
- Tuck your chin to prevent over-arching of the neck.
- Hold for a minute even as you breathe continuously.
- Bring the folded leg down.
- Repeat on the other side.
- Repeat two more times on each side.

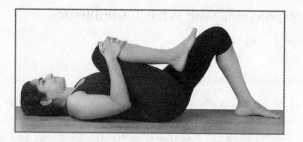

Ardha-Pawanmuktasana with one leg folded

Pawanmuktasana Roll (Roll in the Wind Release Pose)

Stretches the lower back

- Lie down. Take both legs in towards the chest.
- Imprint your back as explained before.
- Hold the legs with one palm on each shin (If you have sensitive knees, hold the thighs).
- Press your thighs in towards the chest.
- As you do that, make sure your tailbone is going towards the floor to create traction at the lower spine.
- Now roll from side to side to give the spine a nice massage.
- Continue as you breathe for 30 seconds.

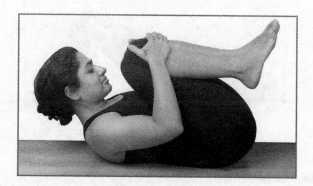

Pawanmuktasana roll

Setu Bandhasana with Pelvic Co-ordination (Bridge Pose)

Restores mobility at hips

- Lie down on the back. Keep the arms comfortably by the side of the hips. You can support your neck and head with a cushion or a rolled towel so that the forehead and the chin are at the same horizontal level.
- Bend your knees so that the feet are flat on the floor, parallel to each other.
- The knees too should be parallel to each other, pointing towards the ceiling.
- Imprint your back as described earlier.
- Maintaining the tone, lift the hips by about three to five inches. Make sure the abs do not jet out.
- Hold the pose as you take three breaths.
- Relax and settle back to the starting position.
- Repeat ten times.

When you press away from the floor, through the shins, the muscles and the connective tissues of the hips and the pelvis stretch, creating a better and deeper connection at the joints.

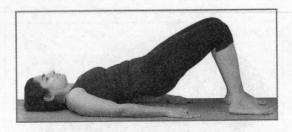

Setu Bandhasana with pelvic tilt

Single Leg Raises

This is the same practice prescribed for knees on page 89 in Chapter

10. Single leg raises also help strengthen the back muscles. If your lower back hurts, make sure you do them with the other leg bent.

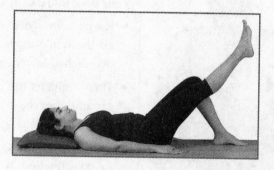

Single leg raise with imprinted back

Side Leg Raises

This is the same practice as the one prescribed for knees on page 90 in Chapter 10. Side leg raises also help strengthen the back muscles. If your lower back hurts, make sure you do them with the lower leg bent.

Marjarasana Breaths on Chair (Cat Pose)

Warms up the spine's postural muscles

- Sit on a chair with a straight back. Make sure your head, neck and spine are in one line on top of each other.
- Place your palms on the knees.
- Through your arms, try to lengthen your back and lift the upper back. This will broaden the upper back and open up the chest. This action should not change the natural curvature of the lower back or overarch it.
- Pull the navel in by an inch or two, feeling the security of the core's support to the lower back.
- Inhale as you expand the chest.
- As you exhale, use the abdominal muscles to push your navel further in towards the lower back. Simultaneously,

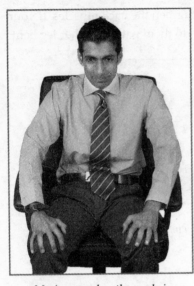

Marjarasana breaths on chair

push the lower back behind, rounding it. This should curve your back into a C.

- Keep your core engaged all the while to prevent an overarched lower back.

- Then inhale to lift and expand the chest, keeping the core engaged.

- Repeat a few times smoothly in coordination with your breaths, without any jerks. It should be a slow, circular pattern to mobilize the back and warm up the muscles of the trunk.

Parvatasana with Wall Support (Mountain Pose with Wall Support)

Stretches the spine

- Stand facing the wall, about six inches away from it, with Tadasana leg alignments, as described on page 82, Chapter 10.

- Place your palms on the wall at waist level.

- Slowly start walking backward while keeping your palms rested on the wall. Walk till your torso and hands are parallel to the floor and the body has made a capital L with reference to the floor.

- Make sure your knees are not locked.

- Take five breaths. Each inhalation expands your chest and presses the four corners of your palm on the wall. Each exhalation takes your belly in and presses the three corners of the feet down on the floor.

- Hold for 30 seconds.
- To release, bend your knees, walk towards the wall and come up.

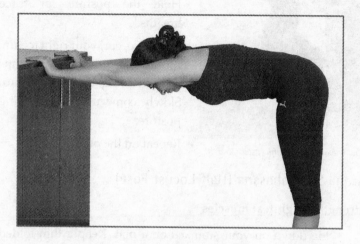

Parvatasana (half) with support

Ashwa Sanchalanasana (Equestrian Pose)

Stretches tight psoas muscles

- Stand with Tadasana leg alignments, as described on page 82, chapter 10.
- Take your right leg behind, toes pointing in front, as much as you can.
- Bring the right knee down.
- Flatten the right toes, such that all toe nails are pressing on the floor.
- Make sure your left knee is on top of your ankle. This is to safeguard the left knee. If the knee goes ahead of the ankle, use your hand to slide your foot forward. Do not bring the leg back to make this adjustment. Such an adjustment will beat the purpose of stretching the psoas muscle.
- Take your hips down as much as possible.

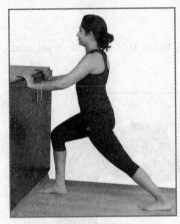

Ashwa sanchalanasana (psoas stretch)

- Lift your torso up. Navel is, of course, pulled in with a gentle squeeze in the hips.

- Hold the posture for three breaths.

- To release, curl your right toes in, lift your knee up, lift your hips up and bring the leg forward. Slowly come up to a standing posture.

- Repeat on the other side.

Ardha Shalabhasana (Half Locust Pose)

Strengthens gluteal muscles

- Lie down on your stomach on a mat. Keep a thin folded blanket under the abdomen if there is lower back strain.

- Rest the forehead on the floor lengthening the neck, without pressing down on the nose.

- Let the hands rest by the side of the body.

- Prepare the body by connecting with your core. Make your legs firm and lengthen the tail bone region.

- Engage the buttock muscles without squeezing them too hard.

- Stretch the right leg, pointing the toes out.

- Lift the right leg straight up from the hip. The lift might not be too high.

- Make sure the right pelvic bone is still on the mat, the right hip pointing down.

- Hold the leg for three breaths.

- Slowly bring it down.

- Repeat on the other side.

- Repeat two more times on each side.

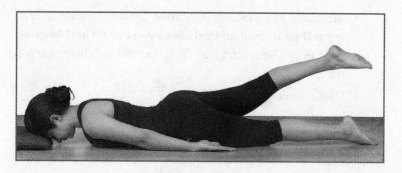

Ardha shalabhasana

Bhujanga-Shalabhasana (Cobra-Locust Pose)

Strengthens back muscles

Let us not get confused with the combination of names and focus instead on safely strengthening the back and the shoulder muscles.

- Lie down on your stomach on a mat. If there is lower back strain, keep a thin folded blanket under the abdomen.
- Rest the forehead on the floor, lengthening the neck, without pressing down on the nose.
- Let the hands rest by the side of the body.
- Prepare the body by connecting with your core. Make your legs firm and lengthen the tail bone region.
- Engage the buttock muscles without squeezing too hard.
- Take your navel in towards your spine.
- Lift the shoulders from the floor without raising the head or the hands from the floor. This is to engage your upper back. Feel the length you create on the sides of the body from your hips to your armpits.
- Inhale and lift the arms, the head and the legs a little off the ground. You will feel like you are extending out from the abs with the lift.

- Maintain this position for three breaths. Inhale as you expand your chest and exhale as you extend and lengthen your upper body and legs. Your breaths will help you feel light.
- Come down gently and relax.
- Repeat three times.

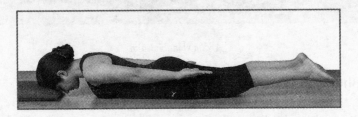

Bhujanga-Shalabhasana

Reverse Walking

Refer to page 158, Chapter 17.
Simple yogic asanas like the ones described in this chapter, when incorporated in our daily routine, ensure relief and protection from painful lower-back conditions.

   Let us now move on to the third area of concern – the upper back-shoulder-neck region.

Chapter 13

BREATHE RIGHT FOR A RIGHT BACK

Breathing involves a continual oscillation between exhaling and inhaling, offering ourselves to the world at one moment and drawing the world into ourselves at the next.
~ David Abram

Did you ever think that how you breathe could affect the health of your back? You will be surprised to learn how much relief proper breathing can bring to backaches!

Back pain is undeniably intertwined with our posture and breathing habits. Muscle imbalances around the spine are the perpetual cause of aches and pains related to the back. For a resilient, pain-free and an injury-resistant back, good posture plays a very important role. Good posture is a symphony of activities involving muscles in the chest, the back, the neck and the abdomen, none as important as the diaphragm. This chapter re-emphasizes the importance of breathing, especially in connection with a healthy lower back.

Diaphragm and Back Pain

A quick revision of what we learned in Chapter 6 on page 44. Our diaphragm lies at the base of our lungs. Exactly beneath the diaphragm are the liver and the stomach. If we breathe primarily by using the muscles attached to our rib cage without taking advantage of the diaphragm's power, we are limiting our breaths. The spine too is intimately connected with the diaphragm. Understanding this symbiotic relationship will steer us in the right direction.

Underuse of the diaphragm causes it to lose strength and forces other muscles to overwork in its place making the entire body compensate. If uncorrected for too long, it makes the body ready for a back injury at the first opportunity. The two most common reasons for an underused and immobilized diaphragm are poor posture and tight abdominals.

Poor Posture

Most of us slump and slouch, and are habitual chest breathers. Therefore, we underuse our diaphragm. When we slump forward, we let the spine round and the head jut forward; the lower ribs dig back and in towards the spine. This compresses the diaphragm and the upper belly. When we sit tall, our lower ribs lift off the abdomen and the adjacent upper belly becomes spacious.

Tight Abdominal Muscles

Tight abdominal muscles too restrict the movement of the diaphragm. If the abdominal muscles do not relax properly, the diaphragm cannot move fully. Stress and fear can lead to gripping in this area, which is usually combined with holding of the breath. These are common habitual responses to anxiety and stress, and who is not stressed these days?

The abdominal muscles need to be strong enough to perform their job. At the same time, they should not be so short, tight and rigid that they restrict lung expansion and limit inhalation.

How Diaphragmatic Breathing Stops Back Pain

Please refer to page 50, Chapter 6 for details on how to adopt diaphragmatic breathing.
Retaining the space our diaphragm needs to move freely is one of the most effective ways to align the spine. It organizes the bones and tones the muscles thus stabilizing the spine from the inside out.

- Every deep diaphragmatic breath pulls on the bones of the lower back, stimulating healthy movement and blood flow around these bones and discs. A strong enough tug can even cause a spinal self-adjustment and optimal alignment.

- A strong diaphragm directly reduces strain and tension in any secondary muscles that may have been inadvertently overworking. This reduces tension in the lower back muscles.

- Diaphragmatic breathing brings the right tone in the abdominal muscles. It keeps our abdominals in optimal working order, training them to relax and lengthen as well as to contract and shorten. This counteraction of every muscle is of utmost importance. By breathing well, it is possible to strengthen the abdominals and yet keep them away from tightness.

- Diaphragmatic breathing acts as a gentle massage for the internal organs. If referred pain from organ discomfort is the cause of lower back pain, stimulating internal movement can reduce those symptoms.

- Diaphragmatic breathing is hard-wired to stimulate the de-stress (parasympathetic) mechanisms in our body. If the cause of a person's lower back pain is stress-related, slow diaphragmatic breathing offers an immediate solution.

Enjoy breathing!

Chapter 14

JACKS IN THE SAME BOX – HEAD, NECK, UPPER BACK AND SHOULDERS

It is not what you look at that matters, it is what you see.
~ Henry David Thoreau

The head is placed on the support of the vertebra of the upper spine in the neck region (cervical). The neck is the most mobile region of the spine. It carries the weight of the head, which is much heavier than the neck itself. The cervical structure leverages a 180-degree, side-to-side movement and also facilitates a forward-backward tilt. This region is as vital as it is precariously poised and requires protection against any injury. Warm, loving support to relax it, whenever possible, is the least we can do to appreciate this impeccable mechanism.

The neck confirms our thought process. A downward nod indicates an affirmation and a side-to-side turn of the neck indicates a no. When in doubt a side tilt is a reflex action. The neck is, literally and figuratively, a junction between the head and the heart. Not only does it allow blood to flow smoothly up to the brain through the major blood vessels situated along its length, it also connects and balances our intellect with our emotions. This deep connect is at its best when the head is well-aligned with the spine. It enables an energized breathing cycle. A 'pain in the neck' is a severe and common phenomenon which can impair concentration and working capacity.

It is not only the neck which emotes; even our arms and hands gesticulate to express thoughts. Humanity's essence is embedded in the hands and the shoulders. Our shoulders too are messengers of our heart – we feel the burden on the shoulders when we are loaded with responsibilities, while strong shoulders indicate a responsible attitude. A shrug expresses doubt and you do feel ignored when you are given a cold shoulder. The movements of our arms express our social intentions – outstretched arms express an open heart, while crossed arms show a closed attitude.

Structure

As we saw in an earlier chapter, the neck's bone structure consists of the cervical spine, the first seven vertebrae. It has a gentle curve and forms a mild C with the bump towards the body.

Bones:

i. Consisting of 12 vertebrae, the thoracic spine is the continuation of the cervical spine in the upper back region. The vertebrae also connect to the ribs, where a breast bone is placed firmly at the front centre of the chest.

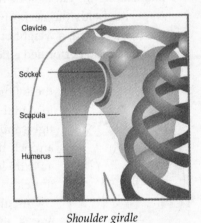

Shoulder girdle

ii. The chest has a framework of 12 pairs of ribs that form a strong cage-like structure to protect the heart and the lungs inside it. This region of the spine is less mobile compared to the lower back or the neck, which do not have a similar bony support.

iii. The shoulder blades (scapulae) are two flat triangular bones present on each side, just behind the rib cage. Many important muscles attach themselves to the scapulae. Reduced scapular movement plays a very important role in upper back, shoulder and neck pain.

iv. The shoulder joint is designed to provide mobility to the arms. It is also prone to dislocation and injuries. The upper end of the arm bone joins the scapulae to make the shoulder joint.

The neck, the shoulders and the upper ribs form the shoulder girdle.

Although there are many muscles in the region, the diamond-shaped trapezius is crucial to keep the head well aligned. It also shapes and strengthens the upper back.

Muscles: The 'Diamond' Muscle

i. Upper Trapezius: This muscle runs from the base of the skull, along the nape of the neck to the shoulders. The upper trapezius holds the neck up in position for hours, carrying the human head, a weight of about four to six kilograms. An amazing task, performed efficiently.

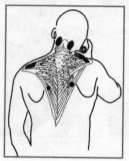

Trapezius muscles

When the head protrudes forward, these fibres are overstrained to carry the load of the head. Eventually, they become tight and get shortened. For every half an inch that our head protrudes, it puts an extra load of 10 kilograms on the poor muscles!

As the upper trapezius constantly works, the nerves that pass underneath squeeze to trigger neck pain, numbness/tingling in the arms, headache, etc.

ii. Lower Trapezius: This muscle secures the scapulae to the upper back and provides a strong foundation for the movement of the arms. The lower trapezius is engaged when the scapulae are pulled behind, close to each other. This also opens the rib cage as the shoulders align correctly in their sockets.

When we round our upper backs, with shoulders rolled forward, the lower trapezius is not used at all. Therefore, they become weak and ineffective, and lead to pain and discomfort in the upper and middle back.

Self-Assessment

By now, we have started enjoying knowing more about our own self. Let us now assess our neck and shoulder region.
Stand with your back towards the wall and let your buttocks lightly brush the wall.

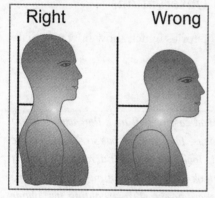

Neck/Head alignment

- Do the shoulders touch the wall?
- Is there more space behind one shoulder than the other?
- Can you touch the back of your head to the wall without arching the neck?
- Is the space between the back of the neck and the wall more than one to two inches?

Now, watch your profile in a mirror.

- Do the shoulders round or lean forward?
- Is one shoulder higher than the other?
- When seen from the front, is the head at the centre or tipped to one side?
- In your side profile, is the head in line with the spine or does it jut forward?

Ideally:

- The shoulders should be relaxed and not stressfully pulled up towards the ears.

- They must not have a rounded contour along the upper back, but should be positioned by the side of the chest.
- The head and the neck should be in a vertical alignment with the body and should not tilt or jut out in front.
- The chin should not point up and should be parallel to the floor.
- The neck has a small concavity, but the head should remain over the spine in the side profile.

Common Observations

Let me share some short case histories which show how we create our own problems.

Stiff Neck

Preeti came to the clinic with a bad case of stiff neck that was limiting her ability to turn her head sideways. The problem was so severe that she would have to turn at her waist to look into the side mirrors of her car. It had become impossible for her to look up without manipulating her spine backward. The problem began the day she started holding her phone handset between her tilted head and a propped up shoulder. What started as a mild attack of a stiff neck turned into an acute case, progressing to the 'frozen' stage.

Head Ahead

Now, take the case of Anil. His job had him working relentlessly at the computer, with his eyes glued and head leaned towards the screen. At the end of the day, he would experience 'hot spots' behind his neck. He had repeated attacks of dull, nagging headaches. The symptoms would subside when he lied down on his back. With deadlines approaching, he worked late into the night. Gradually, he started feeling occasional numbness and a tingling sensation down his arms. Avoiding the use of a pillow while sleeping further aggravated his condition, as his chin would be pushed up. The tightness behind his neck would not permit the muscles behind his neck to stretch into a relaxed position.

I recommended a simple practice called Head Glide, described later on in the chapter, for instantaneous relief to the two problems described here.

Head ahead, if left unattended: When the head often hangs in a forward position, we have to lift our face by arching the neck. This strains the neck muscles and also affects the bones and the soft structures of the joints of the neck. Over time, there is wear and tear of the discs, the cartilages and the nerves, which may lead to compression, reduced blood flow, degeneration and arthritis, a condition called cervical spondylitis. An abnormal, protruded head can cause headaches. As nerves compress due to the disturbed architecture in the region, tingling and numbness in arms may surface.

Rounded Upper Back

A lifestyle of minimal movement encourages the spine to move forward and distorts its S curve into a deep C curve. The rounded upper back, also known as called kyphosis, is the exaggeration of the convexity.

It is a mistake to let the upper back substitute the job of the hips. In activities like tying shoe laces or sitting at the study, we inadvertently use our upper back to reach out for different things by bending forward at the upper back, instead of bending at the hips. In the trade-off, we pay a big price. When the upper back folds forward in a deep C, the muscles in the front of the body pull the skeletal components of the upper body. The scapulae and the shoulders also get pulled forward. As a consequence, the lower trapezius becomes weak.

The head leads the body; so do the arms. The muscles around the shoulders, needed to move and hold the arms in front, work more than the opposing muscles that take the arm behind, or the ones that try to rotate the shoulder open. This imbalance leads to rounded shoulders, as seen from the side. The misalignment of the upper back gives way to a burning sensation in the area between the shoulder blades.

As the joints of the upper torso get pulled forward, they go out of alignment and the circulation in the region gets constricted. This causes numbness and tingling in the shoulders and arms while sleeping or resting. Upper back stiffness prevents you from turning your head even while driving a car.

Harmful effects of slouching

- Height loss: The slouch compresses the upper back by about one to two inches. Regain this height by a simple correction in the posture.

- Increased waistline: Slumping compresses the front of the rib cage at the mid-section to make it wider. This pushes the belly out. Try this: Sit the way you normally do. Measure your waistline. Now, sit tall, breathe deep, pull the navel in slightly and measure the waist at the same point. You have instantly slimmed your waistline by one to two inches!

- Nagging pains and aches: Hot spots in the upper back and tightness around the shoulders are all caused by slouching.

- Angina and heart attacks: A slumped back causes the rib cage to collapse and leads to reduced space in the chest. This in turn leads to improper functioning of the lungs and the heart.

- Shallow breathing and low energy levels: Slumping can reduce the breathing capacity by 20 to 30%, as the rib cage cannot expand in a slouched position. This reduces oxygenation to the whole body, including the brain, and makes a person feel lethargic and fatigued.

- Headaches and migraine: When the brain is deprived of oxygen, it cries out for help, in the form of headaches and migraines. In the forward head position, the muscles adjacent to the blood vessels lock, incapacitating the upward transportation of oxygen-rich blood.

- Tired eyes: For the same reason as mentioned in the previous point, the eye muscles are also deprived of oxygen, and the eyes get tired quickly. This in turn precipitates headaches and migraine.

• Hump behind the neck: Cultural mores force women to hold their breastbone down to conceal the shape of their breasts, as a gesture of modesty. This pulls the collar bones downward and gives an additional pull forward to the head and the neck. The outcome is a strained back part of the neck, where fat and connective tissue start to accumulate as a hump, a condition known as the Dowager's hump. This can be prevented if the rib cage is a little more open, by giving a gentle lift to the breast bones.

Frozen shoulders

The modern movement patterns utilize only 50% of the shoulder functions. Our movements get restricted as we confine ourselves to the chair – at office, at home, in restaurants, in movie halls, almost everywhere.

The underworked shoulders are in a fix when they are suddenly asked to pull out a suitcase from the overhead cargo bin in an airplane, or to take a jar from a top rack. It becomes very challenging as the shoulders have never been subjected to such activity. Even birds confined to cages gradually lose their ability to fly. The moral of this lesson is to maintain a healthy routine of movement and activity, especially for the muscles that are generally kept out of action.

As pointed out earlier, women are socially more prone to develop tension in the shoulder and the chest regions because they do not fold arms behind the head (the way men do) to keep breasts unnoticeable.

Shoulders, unlike other joints of the body, do not have a distinctive pain pattern. Stiffness often takes the shape of pain. It is common to see a patient walk into a clinic with a frozen shoulder that does not hurt, yet refuses to budge beyond a certain point. With the exception of accidents, stiffness or pain in the shoulders is because they are out of their proper position.

Restricted shoulder movements are symptoms of musculoskeletal misalignment that arises when shoulders are deprived of the full range of movements they are designed for. Even simple tasks become very challenging when the shoulders are required to do things they are not used to doing. There is either excruciating pain, or a deeper muscle snaps and tears off.

Necessary Corrections

In order to treat the head, the neck, the upper back and the shoulders as one unit – just as they are meant to be – the following corrections are necessary. The 'Do It Right' sections of this chapter and the strengthening practices described in the next two chapters should help us achieve this goal.

- The shoulder blades should be lowered and pulled behind slightly towards the midline to open the chest. This will comfortably lower the shoulders away from the ears and rotate them slightly outwards.

- The head should be consciously taken back in line with the central axis so that the neck and the shoulder girdle fall into alignment.

- The overused and shortened upper trapezius muscle requires a release through lengthening and intermittent stretching.

- The weakened lower trapezius muscle needs to become stronger to pull the scapulae in place.

- The tight chest and shoulder muscles need regular, healthy stretching.

Do It Right – Head Glide

This practice releases the neck and the shoulders from 'hot spots' and helps the neck muscles at the back relax. To do this, the back of the neck needs to be made long and brought in line with the rest of the spine. Whenever you notice your chin sticking forward and the head leading the body, correct it by applying the following steps. They take only a few seconds but are good enough to cure neck pain and spondylitis.

- Stand or sit straight.

- Gently glide your head back, keeping the chin parallel to the floor.

- Do not over-tip or drop your head back to arch the neck. Instead, the back of your neck should feel elongated.

- Pretend that you are trying to touch the back of your neck to an imaginary wall behind. Or imagine you are wearing a crown like a king or queen, which you love to hold high.

- Avoid the other extreme where, to lengthen the back of your neck, you tilt the chin towards the chest. It is gliding your chin and head behind, and not tucking the chin in.

- In addition, if your tendency is to point the chin up when you sleep on your back, roll two towels to support your neck. This eases the tightness in the neck muscles, bringing joy and comfort.

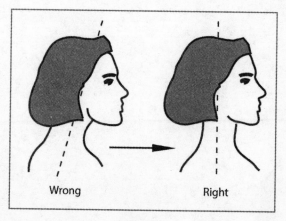

Wrong   Right

Head glide

You will notice that:

- The back part of your neck will feel stretched and the upper back will flatten.

- Your breathing will improve drastically.

Do It Right – Stop the Slouch

- The head glide will flatten your upper back. To stop the slouch:

- Roll your shoulders behind slightly.

- Push the shoulders down away from your ears to lengthen the sides of your neck.

- Your chest will gently move forward to rid the upper back of its slouch.

Chapter 15

HOLD YOUR HEAD HIGH

'Where attention goes, energy flows... and awareness grows.'
~ Anonymous

Muscle-wise, our lifestyle creates an imbalance in the trapezius muscle which supports the neck and upper back from behind. The upper trapezius muscle becomes tight as it has to work very hard to hold the head, while the lower trapezius, is underworked and becomes weak. This pulls the shoulder blades and the shoulders forward. The problem can be dealt with by stretching and relaxing the upper trapezius, and strengthening the lower one. This helps balance the shoulders, the shoulder blades as well as the chest/rib cage. The neck, the head and the spine also all fall in line.

The head, the neck and the upper back are birds of a feather; treating just one is an incomplete answer to the problem affecting the whole area. Yogasanas deal with this zone in totality.

Therapeutic Practices for the Head, the Neck and the Upper Back

Paschima Namaskar / Parsva Hastasana (Namaskar Behind Back)

Opens shoulder joints and chest

The neck and the shoulders are a storehouse of accumulated stress. The easiest way to release this stress is with a namaskar (prayer pose) positioned behind the back. This practice comfortably stretches the wrists and the hands, and also improves the breath.

- You can either sit on the edge of a firm and stable chair or stand with an engaged core. (Refer to page 47, chapter 6. – "Core Stability".)

- Lengthen the spine at the back of your neck, glide your head behind and take the crown of your head away from your body. (Refer to page 136, chapter 14. – "Jacks in the Same Box – Head, Neck, Shoulder and Upper Back".)

- Stretch the arms on the sides like the letter T, palms facing down.

- Rotate the arms inwards. The thumbs point down and the palms turn in further.

- Bend the elbows and bring the lower hands behind the back. The middle fingers touch each other and the little fingers gently press against the back. The fingers point down.

- Gently turn the fingertips upward so that the palms come towards each other to form the namaskar. You can stop midway if you feel that the stretch is enough for you. Breathe while your chest lifts and opens up.

- If the palms comfortably touch each other to form a namaskar, press them more firmly together.

- The head and the spine are in one line and the neck is relaxed. Create length from the pelvic base to the crown of the head.

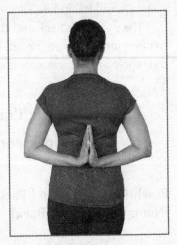

Pashchim namaskar

- Alternative simpler technique:

If due to any pain or restriction, it is not possible to place the palms in the prayer pose on the back, then just fold the arms behind the back and try to hold one elbow or forearm with the other palm. Lift the chest and take deep breaths for a minute. Repeat it with arms crossed the other way.

- Hold your final posture for 15 seconds while you continue to breathe with awareness.

- Repeat three times.

Garudasana Arms (Eagle Pose – Only Arms)

Opens the upper back and shoulder joints

This asana releases tension behind the shoulders.

- You can either sit or stand. Lengthen your spine and engage the abs.

- Stretch your hands out straight in front of you, at shoulder level, palms facing the ceiling.

- Place your right hand over your left hand such that the right upper arm is on the left upper arm.

- Bend both elbows. The backs of both hands now face each other.

- Tuck the right elbow firmly under the left and press the back of the hands against each other.

- If you can go deeper, stretch the back of your shoulders to have the palms face each other with minimal bend at the wrists. The palms will not be at the same level, the fingertips of the left hand will press against the base of the right palm.

- Lift the elbows up as much as you can.

- Push your elbows away from your torso.

- Breathe comfortably and hold the hands for a minute.

- Feel the stretch and softening in your upper back muscles.

- Release gently, step-by-step.

- Repeat with the left arm on top of the right.

- After you are done on both sides, spread your arms on the sides like a T and wrap your arms around the chest, giving yourself a good hug. Walk your fingertips to the shoulder blades and towards the upper spine as much as is comfortably possible.

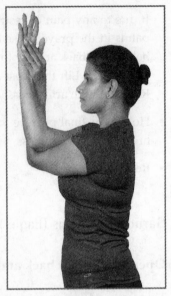

Garudasana arms

- Breathe deep into your upper back and between the shoulder blades.

- Hold for ten seconds.

- Release gently and repeat with the other arm up.

Dwikonasana Arms (Double Angle Pose – only arms)

Stretches muscles in front of the shoulders

The muscles in front of the shoulders are usually tight. This practice strengthens the muscles that extend the shoulders and helps take the shoulder blades in (lower trapezius).

- Stand tall, with the outer edges of the feet parallel and hip-width apart, like in Tadasana. (Refer to page 82, Chapter 10.)

- Lift your chest.

- Lower your shoulders and roll the shoulder blades behind towards each other.

- Take your hands behind you, palms facing each other.

- Interlock the fingers behind your back. If they do not reach, loop a belt around the wrists and hold the belt with the hands as close to each other as possible.

- Keep the elbows slightly bent so that the upper arms go back easily.

- Inhale and lift the chest.

- Pull the arms away from the hips against the resistance of the clasped hands or belt.

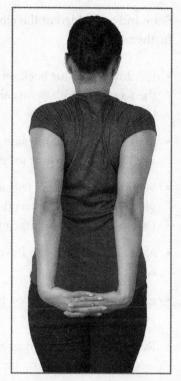

Dwikonasana arms

- Hold the pose for 30 seconds as you breathe with ease.

- Release gently.

- Repeat five times.

Setu Bandhasana (Bridge Pose)

Strengthens entire back, shoulders, thighs and legs

Along with mobilizing the hips, as mentioned in Chapter 12 page 118, the Bridge Pose also has an opening effect on the chest. The tired muscles on the back of the neck get a soothing stretch too. This is a slight variation from the one done for the lower back. Note the position of the hands – the upper arms rest on the floor and are folded at the elbows. This engages the upper back further.

- Lie down on your back on a mat, with the knees folded, and the feet hip-width apart, about six to eight inches away from the hips.

- Place the arms by the side of the body with the palms facing up. Take a few breaths to relax the body.

- With the feet and the legs aligned, press the knees away from you to curl the tail bone down, so that the pelvis stays wide. Do a couple of back imprints. (Refer to page 115, Chapter 12.)

- Now fold the arms on the elbows so that the palms are facing each other.

- Exhale with an imprinted back and lift the hips and the spine off the floor.

- Roll each shoulder closer to the midline so that you feel the weight of your body on top of the shoulders.

- Keep your thighs parallel to each other, point the knees straight forward.

- Feel the gentle tone in the muscles of the buttocks.

- Also feel the stretch in and the lengthening of the neck muscles, the chest and the front of the thighs.

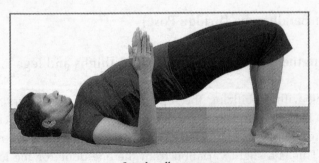

Setu bandhasana

- You can bring your hands down and interlock the fingers underneath your back. Press the arms down for a better lift.

- Continue to breathe well as you hold the posture for 30 seconds.

- Exhale softly, release the arms first, and then gradually bring the upper back, the middle back and the lower back down vertebra by vertebra.

- Repeat five times.

Simpler Techniques

Strengthen muscles behind the shoulders.

Due to pain or any restrictions, if performing the preceding practices is difficult, there is a simple alternative. The following set of four exercises beautifully engages and strengthens the upper back muscles. We call it the 'T-W-Puppet-aaaa' sequence. After practising these for a few weeks, you can move on to the practices listed earlier.

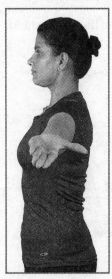

T arms

i. T Arms

- Whenever you feel your shoulders have rolled in front causing your upper back to round, freshen the upper back region with this practice.

- In a well-aligned standing pose, raise your arms horizontally at the level of your shoulders, to form the letter T.

- Bend your elbows gently.

- With palms open and facing the front, point the thumbs up. Ensure that your head is rightly aligned over the body. (Refer to page 136, Chapter 16.)

- Initiating the movement from the upper back, turn the palms up towards the ceiling and roll them behind. Roll the thumbs behind and down as much as possible.

- Press shoulders down, away from the ears.

- While holding this arm position, notice how the scapulae or the shoulder blades come closer to the midline (lower trapezius action).

- Take four long breaths as you hold the pose.

- Release the shoulder blades by turning the thumbs up.

- Repeat ten times.

ii. W Arms

- Bend the arms at the elbow as if you are making a W with your arms.

- The shoulders are lowered, away from the ears.

- The elbows are at a level lower than the shoulders.

- Lift the chest and the rib cage up and push the arms behind. This action engages the lower trapezius.

- Take four long breaths as you hold the pose, and release.

- Repeat ten times.

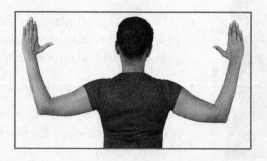

W arms

iii. Puppet Arms

- Lie down comfortably on your back.

- You may keep your legs folded at your knees.

- Raise both your hands straight up, palms facing each other.

- Raise your right hand straight up at the shoulder and tuck it back in the socket, in a puppet-like movement.

- Repeat on the other side.

- Continue alternate raise-and-tuck of arms.

- Breathe normally as you do the practice for about a minute or for 30 counts on each side.

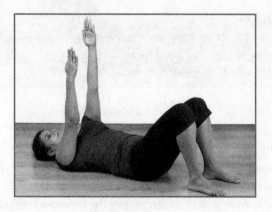

Puppet arms

iv. Arm Raises with 'aaaa' Chants

- Lie down as in the earlier practice.

- Keep your entire back in contact with the floor.

- You may keep your knees bent, especially if you have a sensitive lower back.

- Inhale as you stretch your hands out on the floor at shoulder level, palms facing up.

- Exhale; chant a nice and long 'aaaa' as the hands come up parallel to each other, palms facing each other. Make the chant last through the movement and the movement last through the chant. The chant ensures that your exhalations are long and the practice is slow.

- Elbows are straight and soft through the practice.

- Bring the hands down slowly.

- Repeat the arm raises ten times, with breath control and chants.

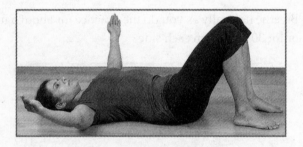

Arm raises with 'aaaa' chants

Once you are able to do this sequence comfortably, you can add the exercises mentioned at the beginning of this chapter to strengthen you upper back further.

These simple practices can relieve the tense and stiff shoulders and the muscles of the upper back. Spend about 10-15 minutes twice a day doing these exercises and reap the benefits all through the day.

Having gone through the postural alignments of all the major joints of the body, I would now like to take you through a few exercises that can be done during the day – a much needed break; especially if you have a desk job that requires you to sit in one place for hours together.

Chapter 16

ANYTIME ANYWHERE STRETCHES

Life is like riding a bicycle. To keep your balance,
you must keep moving.
~ Albert Einstein

The human body is designed to be physically in motion; there is no room for lethargy and long, sedentary spells. In spite of this knowledge, man indulges in comforts and luxuries. Studies have shown that musculoskeletal back problems are the largest cause of disability among working people and that 30% of these problems become chronic.

Sitting with an elongated back and neck, without a forward or backward tilt, makes for a graceful posture. But, however graceful and attractive a posture be, it is important to remember to avoid sitting for more than thirty minutes in the same position. Find a good reason, or a flimsy one, for a refreshing break. A couple of minutes off, perhaps just to say a casual hello to a workmate or to have a sip of water. This small break nourishes the body and the mind. Smile without a reason, feel good about yourself, and watch the stress levels deplete and the breaths become calm and harmonious. These feel good tips do not cost money or time; only your positive intention!

Practising right workplace ergonomics to correct the posture is an effective way to work energetically. Some specific exercises for the neck and the back can further improve the posture and the personality.

Stretch the Body, Stretch the Mind

For a positive and cheerful outlook at work, remember to be kind to the neck and the spine. Encourage the movements they are designed for. This may keep even the Monday morning blues at bay. Sometimes a grumpy, irritable, frowning attitude may be due to low-intensity discomfort in the neck region.

- It is recommended that you take a five minute break every hour or so.

- A variety of exercises have been described here to address various problems that people generally have. You can pick the ones you need for your specific issue.

- You can set up a routine where you do a few different ones at each break, without letting the number of exercises overwhelm you. Do whatever and how much ever you can and reap the benefits.

- For each exercise, hold the posture at its final position for ten seconds. Release and repeat each exercise ten times. This way, you can pick three exercises for each five-minute break.

- Breathe mindfully when you maintain a pose. Do not hold your breath at any time.

Office Practices for Neck, Upper Back and Shoulders

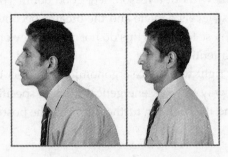

Wrong – Chin jutting   *Right – head glide*

Head Glide

Aligns the head, the neck and the upper back
- Refer to page 136, Chapter 14.

Neck Stretch

Stretches the muscles at the sides of the neck

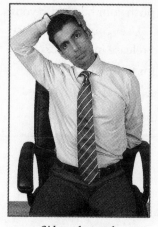

- Do the head glide, as mentioned before.
- Hold the left side of your forehead with your right hand.
- Gently pull the head to the right side.
- Feel a comforting stretch along the left side of the neck.
- Hold the position for three breaths.
- Release gently.
- Repeat on other side.

Side neck stretch

- Repeat two more times on both sides.

T Arms

Corrects rounded shoulders and the 'hot spot' sensation in the upper back
- Refer to page 145, Chapter 15.

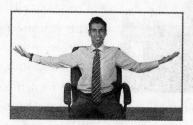

T arms

Head Press

Releases strain in the neck

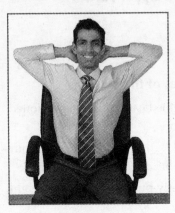

Head press

- Interlock your hands behind your head, palms facing the head.
- Press the head against the resistance of the hands as you try to push your head with your hands. Use counter-resistance to find release in the neck.
- Hold for ten counts.
- Release and repeat ten times.

Elbow Press

Tones the upper back

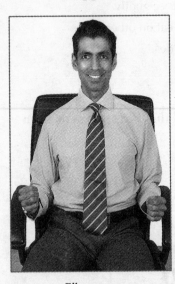

Elbow press

- Sit tall on your chair facing a table.
- Place your elbows on the table such that the palms face each other, while the fingers and the thumbs point towards the ceiling.
- Make sure your neck and shoulders are relaxed.
- Press your elbows on the table.
- This will lower your shoulders, increasing the distance between them and your ears.
- Hold for ten counts to engage the upper back.
- Release and repeat ten times.

Chair Press

Tones the lower back and the core and strengthens the back

This is an instant lower back and belly strengthening practice for those with an overarched lower back and weak abdominals.

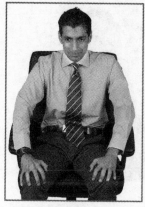

- Sit tall on a chair.
- Make sure that your bottom is touching the back of the seat.
- As you exhale, pull the belly button in and let your lower back make full contact with the back of the seat.
- Hold for ten counts.
- Release and repeat ten times.

Chair press

Therapeutic Spinal Stretches

Side bends

Loosen and strengthen the spine on either side

- Slide to the edge of the chair and sit upright.
- Interlock the fingers and lift the arms over your head.
- Keep the elbows straight, turn the interlocked palms upwards to face the ceiling.
- Push up your wrists rather than just the fingers.
- The breathing will now be deep and invigorating.
- As you exhale, slowly bend to one side and feel the stretch.
- Make sure the upper side of your body does not leaning forward.
- Hold the position for ten counts.
- Inhale as you come back to the centre.

- Repeat on the other side.
- Repeat the cycle three more times.

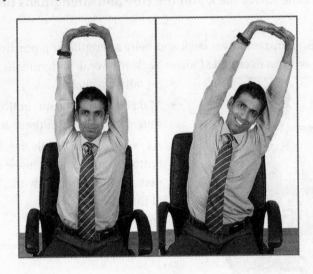

Side bends

Partial Forward Bend – Parvatasana with Wall Support (Mountain Pose with Wall Support)

Lengthens and stretches the spine.

- Refer to page 121, Chapter 12.

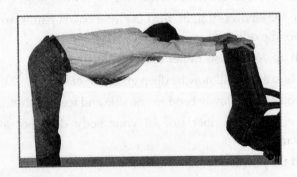

Partial forward bend

Back Bend

Expands the chest and reverses the slouch

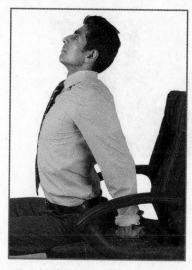

- Sit tall at the edge of a chair.
- Place the fingertips of your hands on the seat, just behind your hips.
- Inhale and elongate the spine.
- Let the navel get pulled in as you lift the chest up.
- Hold for ten counts.
- Release and repeat three more times.

Back bend

Chair Twist

Releases stiff back

- Sit on a chair, with one side of your body towards the back of the chair.
- Hold the back of the chair with both your hands at the chest level.
- Twist from the waist.
- Lengthen the spine and deepen the twist.
- Make sure your navel is tucked in and is pointing towards the back of the chair.
- Hold the stretch for ten counts.
- Release and repeat on the other side.
- Repeat two more times on both sides.

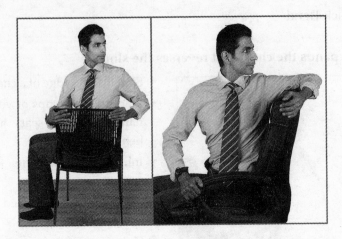

Chair twists

Tone Tonic

Whenever you get a chance or whenever you realise that your muscles have gone loose, bring some tone in them. Your mantras are:

1. **Navel In** (Refer page 47, chapter 6.)

2. **Clench the hips** (Refer page 48, chapter 6.)

Focused Mindful Breathing

You can relax any tense muscle by breathing slow and deep, with the entire focus on the tight zone.

- As you inhale through the nose, imagine you are inhaling into the area where your muscles feel tight or uncomfortable. It could be your neck, the upper back, or the waist region.

- As you exhale through the nose, imagine you are breathing out through the pores of the same area. Consciously relax the area as you feel all the tension release with the exhalations.

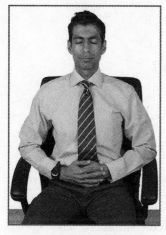

Mindful breathing

- Take a few breaths in this manner. You might feel the discomfort increase in the first few breaths. But soon enough, you will sense a release.

Intermittent stretches while on the chair, or what we call office yoga – frequent breaks, small walks in the office, wriggling the toes, rotating the ankles, flexing and stretching the knees, side-to-side hip movement, shoulder rotations, facial massage with warm palm – goes a long way in maintaining good posture. Run your hands lightly over the tired calves, thighs, abs, back, shoulders, neck, face and head. This can be an endearing experience while sitting on the chair itself. The best part is that nobody around will even suspect that you have had a complete postural work out. They will only see the result in a fatigue-free you.

Chapter 17

REVERSE WALKING

If at first the idea is not absurd, then there is no hope for it.
~ Albert Einstein

Whenever you encounter a difficult situation, 'take a step back'. So goes an oft-repeated advice. Good advice. Taking that step back boosts your capability to deal with tough times. In fact, actual, physical backward locomotion is proving to be a powerful trigger to mobilise physiological resources for better health, that is, better blood sugar control in diabetics, balanced hormones and a stronger immunity.

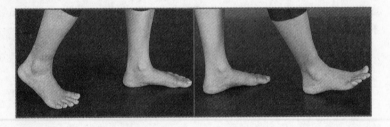

Reverse walking – Toe strike   *Forward walking – Heel strike*

A common saying in the Eastern cultures is: To extend your life span with good health, do backward exercises. At public parks in China, it is common to witness many people walking backward, as a form of exercise. Retro-exercise or retro-running has been popular for many years in Europe.

Reverse walking is a good exercise to reduce stress in any part of the body. When you go backwards, your stomach works out like your back and creates a nice reaction for your abdominals.

Walking or jogging every day is recommended for a healthy lifestyle; but they can be too time – consuming, making it difficult to be regular at the exercise. The good news is that:

- A hundred steps of backward walking are equivalent to a thousand steps of conventional walking.

- Ten minutes of backward walking have the same benefits as more than an hour of forward walking.

- Backward walking does not require a lot of space. You can do it anywhere – in your backyard or on the terrace of your office building, during snack time.

How to Begin?

- Start gradually along a row of tiles in a spacious area in your home or on the terrace. It is advisable not to go out on the road so as to avoid potholes, sign boards, cars and other hazards.

- Let the pace be slightly slower than your normal forward walking speed.

- Make sure you are not flaying your feet outward while you walk. That is, your feet should land parallel to each other and not form a V.

- After reaching the end of the room, turn and walk in reverse all through.

- Gradually increase the time from 5 minutes to 10-15 minutes, twice a day.

- As you feel more comfortable, increase your speed gradually to that of your normal forward walking pace.

- But do keep an eye out for where you are going – safety first!

Where and Why Does Reverse Walking Work?

Better cardio-respiratory fitness

At a given pace, an athlete can increase the heart rate to 156 beats per minute with backward walking as compared to 106 beats with forward walking. This develops endurance and eventually helps reduce elevated blood pressure. The heart and the lungs get a better workout too with this form of exercise.

Increased energy expenditure

Walking backward burns several times more calories than jogging. Muscle (electromyographical) activity of the lower extremities is greater in backward versus forward walking, which suggests that at a similar pace, you can expend more energy in a shorter period of time.

Increased metabolism

The leg muscles work in a different manner when you reverse walk, activating an otherwise sluggish metabolism. Backward walking technically triggers a concentric contraction (shortening) of your quadriceps (front thigh muscles). This type of contraction is a metabolically expensive movement, which means it burns a lot more calories compared to eccentric movement (lengthening) of the thigh muscles, involved in walking forward.

Better brain and balance

Walking backward is a neurobic activity that causes new neural connections to grow in your brain. This happens because reverse walking involves one or more of your senses in a novel context. Since you cannot see what you are walking into, the other senses sharpen to protect you. It brings better balance, meaning that the vision and the hearing power increase too. It engages your attention and breaks a routine activity in an unexpected way.

Rehabilitation of Lower Extremities – Hips, Lower Back, Knees

You can benefit from working out in reverse even if you are recovering from certain knee or leg injuries, as it puts less stress on the knee joints. Backward travel is unmatched for those who suffer from muscle injuries of the hip, the groin, the hamstrings or the lower back, and can also work for those undergoing post-surgical knee joint rehabilitation.

When you walk backward, the front of your foot strikes the floor first as compared to the heel, unlike in regular walking. Since the direction of the force on the knee joint is reversed, it may help anyone who experiences pain ascending or descending the stairs or hills, or anyone who undergoes pain when performing lunges or squats.

Section IV

REUNITE

The time is always right, to do anything that is right
~ Martin Luther King

Chapter 18

STAND TALL

*The mind's first step to self-awareness must be
through the body.*
~ George A Sheehan

A correct standing posture has the spine stacked vertically, vertebra over vertebra with the correct curvatures. The back and the neck stay elongated and upright. The weight-bearing joints stand precisely vertically on top of each other, coupled with healthy feet and leg alignments. Together, these make standing comfortable and pain-free.

Standing: The Right Ways

Correct standing posture involves following the rules that we now discuss. Some of these have been explored in the previous chapters too.

Parallel Feet

- Stand with your feet at hip-width distance (distance between your ears).

- The outer edges of the feet should be parallel to each other. Most of us habitually stand with the front part of our feet turned significantly out. To nullify the harmful effects of our habits and to activate our weaker inner leg muscles, we must stand with the front part of the feet (toes) turned in by just half an inch. This feels good as it offers stability and balance.

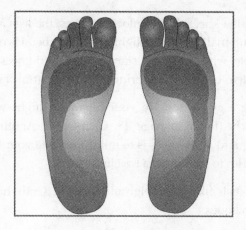

Parallel feet

Strengthened Arches of the Feet

- Prevent rotation of your feet. To do so, do not let your ankles fall in towards the body's midline as it collapses the arches of the feet. Instead, keep your feet parallel to each other as mentioned earlier.

- Press the mounds of your toes down.

- Raise your toes and spread them out. Observe the strength in the arches. Place the toes down.

- Divide the body weight on the three weight-bearing points of the feet. (Refer to page 66, Chapter 8.)

Unlocked Knees

While standing, we tend to put maximum weight on our heels. This pushes the knees back into an overarch and locks the knee joints. This is extremely harmful for the health of the knees. To avoid this:

- Spread the body's weight evenly over the triangular base of the soles – the first and the fifth toes and the heels – and relax the knees. With unlocked knees, the legs are straight but internally soft and slightly bent (the bend is not visible). People, who habitually stand with locked knees, will have to micro-bend them to bring back the neutral state.

- Bring a gentle tone to your hips and thighs with a Hip Clench. (Refer to page 48, Chapter 6.) Another way to safeguard your knees is to mildly activate your front thigh muscles to give them a baseline tone.

- This feels like your thigh muscles are gently hugging the thigh bones.

- The tone slightly pulls the kneecaps up, thus preventing the knees from getting locked. At the same time, use your thigh muscles to hold your body up instead of weighing down on the joints.

Navel In

This is the same inner corset tone we spoke about in Chapter 6 on page 47.

This would feel like you are zipping your trouser. To recapitulate:

- The navel must be pulled in by a mere half inch towards the back.

- It should not be too tight. Make sure you do not hold your breath.

- In fact, the navel pull should comfortably enhance the breathing.

Small Hollow in the Lower Back

The idea is to avoid the tendency to arch the back. In such cases:

- Imagine you have a tail.

- Now, pull this imaginary tail down towards the heels.

- This should be done with straight but not hyperextended knees. The knees should not bend too much either.

- The belly should not bulge out.

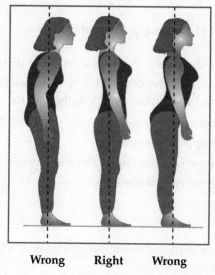

Wrong   Right   Wrong

Standing postures

Vertical Pull

Now that you are well-balanced on your feet:

- Lift the breastbone and the rib cage up without an excessive arch in the lower back. It should feel like a puppeteer has pulled your torso up on a string. This creates a good distance from the hipbone to the rib cage.

- Another way to understand this position well is to employ a good old technique. Place a flat book on the crown of your head and walk. This will help you find the plumb-line (Refer to page 35, Chapter 5.) and create awareness of any habitual or excessive wrong movements that pull you out of alignment.

- When you stand, push your head upward as if there were a light weight on it.

- This technique contracts the neck muscles at the front and gives a stretch to the tight muscles behind the neck. Your neck will actually become longer.

Lowered and Opened-Up Shoulders

- Lower your shoulders, that is, increase the distance between your ears and your shoulders. This has the dual effect of easing the tension in the shoulders and lengthening the cervical spine.
- Rotate the arms gently behind. This opens up the chest and engages the upper back muscles.
- The palms now face the thighs and the thumbs point forward instead of being turned inwards.

Head Glide

We have already explored this technique on page 136, Chapter 14. Let's do a quick recap:

- Pull your head and neck in line with the rest of your spine.

- Take your chin in slightly to make it parallel to the floor.

- The highest point of your body should be the tip of your head from behind.

- Let your breaths become smoother and efficient with a chin tuck.

- Relax the jaw and the neck muscles.

- If you happen to clench your teeth, rest your tongue gently at the roof of your mouth. This automatically relaxes the jaw, which in turn eases any strain on the neck.

    Retain this healthy position from feet to toes, whenever you remember to do so, while comfortably breathing. The ears, the shoulders, the hips, the knees and the ankles will fall in one straight line. However, if this does not occur due to an overarched back or neck, exercises should be added to stretch the shortened muscles and strengthen the weaker ones, as prescribed in earlier chapters.

Instant Alignment Technique

Follow these primary alignment steps as a routine:

- **Toes In, Heels Out** – Stand with the outer edges of your feet parallel to each other.

- **Knees Unlocked** – Keep your knees soft and do not push them behind.

- **Hip Clench** – Bring a gentle tone to your hips by squeezing them mildly.

- **Navel In** – Pull in the abdomen gently and push the lower back slightly behind.

- **Shoulders Down** – Lower the shoulders as you slightly hinge them backwards.

- **Head Glide** – Retract the head to keep the chin parallel to the ground.

Developing the habit of properly aligning the body takes times. It is a prerogative and adhering to its principles is the best thing one can do for the self. 'Practice makes perfect.' Learning to hold the aligned position for some time, each time, will unfold a success story. Slowly, but surely, correct alignments will turn into a habit. Take short creative breaks between these alignment cycles; soon the inner muscle memory will take over as the examiner and the results will be astounding.

Chapter 19

WALK SMART

The less effort, the faster and more powerful you will be.
~ Lao-tze

Walking should not be a lethargic drag for the lower limbs; it should be a series of energetic propulsions. When the leg and the buttock muscles contract strongly to propel the body forward, they are well exercised. This spares the back of unnecessary wear and tear. The buttocks, the legs and the feet do the work, while the torso is stable and moves forward smoothly. The overall sensation should be that of an energetic, lithe glide through space.

A healthy walk retains the centre of gravity in place. Just try to walk with rounded shoulders and a hunched upper back or with a protruded abdomen. This kind of a walk overworks some muscles and puts more pressure on the back and the legs. The centre of gravity shifts from the centre of the body. Try this now; Walk with a book or a bag of grocery (sugar, rice, pulses) on the head. Experience the 'forces' of the core muscles that render a confident gait.

Walking: The Right Ways

The correct manner of walking involves following certain rules. Let us now explore these rules one by one.

Head Up: As you walk, imagine you are suspended from a helium balloon.

- This makes the top of the head move up instead of leaning forward.

- This spot lift keeps the chin from leading the walk.

- It allows the spine to assume more natural curves.

- It also keeps the ears in a more normal position – over the shoulders.

Lightened Walk: Adding a soft tone to the hip muscles (gluts) ensures a healthy and smart walk.

- It prevents the side-to-side hip-rock.

- It smartly moves the forward foot's pelvis.

- It also keeps us in better balance.

- The hip tone helps engage the belt muscle as the navel gets tucked in naturally.

- It supports the lower spine and aligns the pelvis while walking.

Step on a Wider Heel: When we walk, we thrust our body weight on the heel at the point it touches the ground, that is, at the edge of the heel.

- Try landing on the surface of the entire heel rather than only on its rear edge.

- By landing on the entire area of the heel, we engage the foot's spring system.

- This spreads the shock distribution of the landing evenly.

- It prevents strain on the feet and the back.

Reduce the Heel Lift of the Foot Behind: As you land on a wider area of the heel of the foot in front, let the back part of the heel of the foot behind remain in contact with the ground for a fraction of a second before lifting it up. Sounds difficult as we are in motion!

Let me put it this way: When you walk, lift the heel of the foot behind only slightly. We tend to lift that heel up by two to three inches. Try to minimize this lift to just an inch.

This stretches the rear leg and activates the muscles behind the legs in a chain reaction – from the sole up through the buttocks, across to the spine. At this point, the calf muscles are stretched to propel the body forward.

Push Off From the Foot Behind: This is very important to prevent a drag when you walk.

- Activate the foot and the leg behind rather than the ones in front.

- Push off from the toe mounds of the foot behind rather than permitting a passive drag.

- This healthy push off increases the efficiency of getting the leg forward and tones the buttocks in a way no other exercise can.

Gently Swing the Arms: An ideal walk allows for a free and natural swing to the arms. There is neither a need to exaggerate the swing nor to restrict the arms.

- Let the hands be relaxed, without clenched fists.

- A natural arm swing improves the efficiency of motion.

- It allows for a swifter gait, with balanced weight on the legs.

This movement happens naturally when we release the shoulder muscles and relax the upper back by lowering the muscles of that region. This does not mean we slump or round our shoulders. All that we need to do is gently lower the shoulders to encourage a healthy lift of the sternum or the breast bone, without an overarched lower back.

Relax the Jawline: Try to smile with your lower jaw clenched up tightly. The effect is so artificial! Note that we usually keep the lower jaw lifted up. A gentle smile relaxes the lower jaw and the facial muscles too. More important, it releases undue tightness in the head and the neck muscles.

Stride with Ease

In an effort to walk correctly, do not walk hard. Learn to enjoy it. Try these simple and practical methods to move, with alignment.

- Tone the buttocks with a mild squeeze and it will take care of most aspects of a correct walk.

- The pelvis should not swing side-to-side when we walk. Toning the gluteal muscles ensures a better push off from the front part of the feet, rather than a lazy drag.

- Walk like a king or a queen. Imagine you are wearing a crown. What a regal feeling! Not only will you see yourself confident, you will also love the entire experience.

Walking is a fascinating exercise, which burns calories and keeps the muscles fruitfully engaged. You can walk alone or in company; what is important is to enjoy it with a smile.

Chapter 20

SIT STRAIGHT

May we become aware of the truth within
~ Eckhart Tolle

We move our body through a myriad of patterns. A good pattern of movements is an integral part of a good posture. While moving your body to sit on a chair, observe the action. Is there a thud down or slump into the chair? If so, this is because the hip and the knee muscles are relaxed and are not supporting the body the way they are meant to. You would also notice the neck and the lower back getting rounded, outside the safe range of movement.

Height of the Chair

By adjusting its height, every chair can be made ergonomic.

Thighs Parallel to Floor: The height of the chair should be such that the feet rest on the floor and the thighs are parallel to the floor.

For Tall People: Tall people are prone to backaches if they sit on low chairs as the pelvis tilts back to round the lower back and the lower spine gets over-flexed beyond its safe range. Tall people should keep a cushion on the chair and sit on it to elevate the hips and bring them at knee level in the seated position.

For Shorter People: When a short person with a big belly sits on a chair, the pelvis tilts forward, increasing the arch of the lower back. The pressure on the discs and the nerves results in back ache. Such people should use a foot rest and lean against the back of the chair to avoid a slouch.

Judge Ideal Height of Chair: To avoid pain induced by a mismatch between your body and the furniture, do the following. Stand in front of the chair and adjust the height so that the seat is approximately at knee level. A chair that is very high will promote unhealthy postures. In such cases, it is best to sit on the front edge of the chair.

Use Cushion as Necessary: If your lower back overarches or your back rounds when you sit, take a cushion under your hips to avoid either of the wrong curvatures.

Using Core Muscles to Sit

Straighter Back: When you are in the motion of sitting down, avoid bending too much; instead, land your hips with a straighter back on the front part of the chair like in the 'latrine squat'. Then ease yourself to the back of the chair till the spine is comfortably supported by the chair's backrest without rounds or slumps.

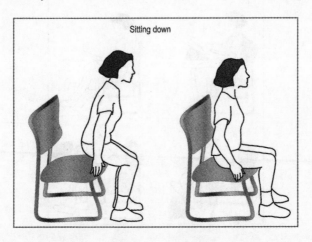

Right way to sit down

Sit on Sitting Bones: Usually, we sit with our upper back slouched behind on the chair, while our hips slide forward. This rounds the lower back. Become aware of the extra load the lower back is subjected to, as the sitting bones are not utilized. Sitting on our sitting bones/hip bones releases the lower back of this pressure. However, in this slouched position, it is not possible to find the sitting bones. To find the sitting bones:

- Sit straight.

- Rock the body side-to-side as if trying to crush the seat of the chair with the hips.

- Feel two bony projections. These are the sitting bones.

- Be conscious to use them when you sit.

- Make sure not to pressurize the lower back.

- Evenly distribute the weight between the two sides. Unknowingly, many of us sit with a slight tilt to one side. Let us become aware of this and push the other side down to distribute the weight evenly.

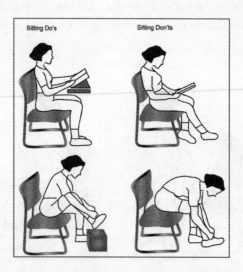

Sitting dos and don'ts

Feet on the Floor

- The feet should rest on the floor with a 90-degree or more bend both at the knees and at the hips.

- Do not sit with the knees crossed.

- Make sure your feet are placed far enough from the chair such that the thighs make a 90-degree angle or more with your lower legs.

- If your hips go lower than the knees, take a cushion below your hips.

- If your hips are a little higher than your knees, it is okay. Just make sure your belly is tucked in so that your pelvis is tilted appropriately.

- If the thighs are too high, which is very unlikely, you need to find a different chair.

  Pelvic Tilt: A healthy seated posture on a chair would mean that our vertebrae are stacked over a correctly placed pelvis. As we discussed in Chapter 11 on page 106, the human pelvis is designed to slightly tip forward. A tilted pelvis allows the spine to stack well over it. We can then remain both upright and relaxed without additional muscle tension to support the bones.

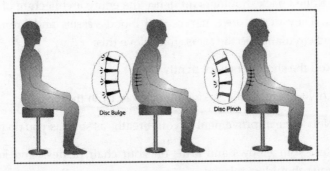

Right   Wrong – Rounded slumping   Wrong – Overarched back

Sitting postures

S Back: All the three normal curvatures of the back should be present when you sit on a chair. Remember not to arch the back beyond the comfort zone, nor to sit with a rounded spine.

- Sit up straight with the back gently stretched up.

- The buttocks should touch the back of the chair.

- If the knees are too close to the chair, blood circulation is affected. So, there should be a gap between the front edge of the chair and the folds of your knees. The gap should be enough to fit in a clenched fist.

- Adjust the back rest of the chair such that you can sit straight.

Belly Magic: As always, keep your belly button pulled in by just half an inch. Loss of muscle tone in the belly region is the main cause of all backaches. The abdominal muscles form the prime support to the spine from the front. The comfort of sitting on a chair has snatched away this dynamic muscle of its tone. A conscious effort to regain it is a must.

Repositioned Shoulders: People with hunched shoulders/ rounded upper backs tend to correct their hunch by pushing the belly forward. This overarches the back. Excessive lumbar curvature with an upright upper body is bound to cause problems.

Rolled back shoulders influence the entire architecture of the area. They decompress nerves and blood vessels and improve blood circulation to the arms. To achieve this:

- Roll the shoulders back gently.

- Lower them a little, taking them away from the ears.

- Notice the improvement in your breaths as soon as you do this.

- Rest your elbows and arms on your chair or desk and keep your shoulders relaxed.

Head Glide: Just like a gentle yet constant tuck in the belly, the head too should always be gliding in, to make the back of the neck long. The chin is parallel to the earth – neither jutting ahead of the body nor pressed down towards the chest. This brings the neck in line with the spine the way it is meant to be. Lengthening the neck is as important as lengthening the back, as it brings tone to the neck muscles. This technique too improves the breathing.

Another technique is to place a flat, light weight object on the head and to moderately push the neck up against it to realign the jawline.

Sitting correctly burns more calories. As we know already, well-toned postural muscles increase metabolism, whereas lax and toneless muscles reduce metabolism and encourage the body's tendency to store fat. By sitting with proper postural alignment and maintaining a balanced tone, we automatically burn more calories.

Getting Up from a Chair

Very often, when we get up from a chair, we do so with a jerk. This should be avoided at all costs. Follow these simple steps every time you get up to minimize or prevent lower back and knee pain.

- When you are ready to get up, move forward to the front of the chair.

- Place your palms gently on your knees.

- If it is not already done, tuck your belly in by half an inch.

- Get up with as straight a back as possible, that is, minimize the forward-lean on your back when you get up.

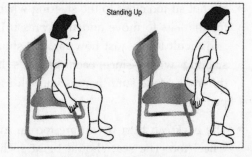

Right way to get up from a chair

Extra Precautions While Driving

The fundamentals of sitting well-aligned in the car must be adhered to diligently. First and foremost, adjust the seat to make the back vertical. This position gives the back a strong support and allows the head to rest against the headrest at the level of the chin.

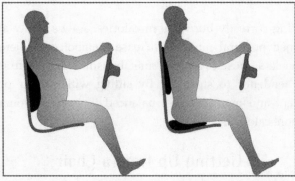

Wrong for overarched back   *Right way to sit on a cushion*

- Knees should be bent at the level of the hips or higher than the hips to reach the pedals. The angle between the thighs and the lower legs should be 90-degrees or more.

- Your upper body should make an angle of about 100-degrees with your thighs (slightly leaned behind). This angle should certainly not be less than 90-degrees.

- Do not sit too close to the steering wheel as it leaves no room for the legs to move and thus pressurizes the lower back. It is difficult to say just how far you should sit away from the steering wheel since each person's body proportions are different. Make sure there is enough room to freely press the pedals.

- The back can hurt if you are too far away from the steering wheel too. The seat should be at such a distance that your knees have a soft bend.

- Sit on a thin cushion. This gives a gentle lift to the hips, relaxes the taut muscles and eases the pressure on the back.

- With the hands on the wheel, the elbows should be slightly bent and relaxed. Avoid shoulder shrugs or rounded shoulders. The same mechanism of lowered and pulled back shoulders comes into play while standing, sitting or walking.

Supports for the Back

We are inclined to use supports behind the back for mechanical support, not knowing that this is not the solution.

Disadvantages of Special Lumbar Support

A lumbar support is a special cushion that attaches to the back rest of a chair or a car seat to create a curvature in the back. People with flat lower backs get the necessary curvature with its push without having to use the muscles needed for this action. So, when they are not using the lumbar support, the spine goes back into unhealthy alignments. This causes damage since wrong muscles stretch with the external pressure of the support. Those who already have an increased arch in their lower back land up with an exaggerated curvature. Therefore, the best support to rely on is our own muscles.

Magic of Sitting on a Simple Cushion

Years of unhealthy sitting habits lead to permanent alteration of muscles and tissues of the surrounding region. The muscles of the hips and the hamstrings become tight and short, while those of the buttocks go weak and stay underdeveloped. To compensate for these distortions, it is beneficial to sit on a support rather than having one behind you, especially when you drive.

- Just like when you sit on a chair, you can use a cushion when you drive too. The support of a cushion raises the hip region and helps to consciously align the pelvis.

- Those with a flat lower back can raise their chest gently to tip the pelvis forward and make sitting an enjoyable experience.

- The spine stacks automatically on the support, so you can sit comfortably for a long time without hurting your back.

- Those with a swayback can also have tight muscles in the front part of the hips, which are used to bend the hips. Sitting on a cushion gives a lift to the trunk and increases the angle of the hip joint, improving the local blood circulation. There is no need to tip the pelvis forward as it is already tipped. It is advisable to engage the abdominals into a healthy tone while sitting on the cushion.

Use of a cushion as a prop is very useful until we have trained the body to use the muscles in the correct way. A good alternative to using a cushion is to sit on the front edge of a firm and stable chair, allowing the pelvis to tip forward.

Advantages of sitting on a cushion:

- Allows you to sit comfortably for hours.

- Makes back muscles relaxed.

- Facilitates better breathing.

- Encourages better circulation in the back.

- Allows for repair and optimum functioning of the abdominal organs.

During the day, frequently check your posture on the chair. With all this knowledge, we no doubt start by sitting up straight, but it is only human to slip back into our habitual, unhealthy postures. This is because the body is used to this comfort zone and demands it. The muscles too love the lethargic attitude since toned muscles involve discipline and effort. However, as you begin repositioning the body alignment every once in a while, with a little effort and awareness, sitting straight will soon become a way of life.,

Gravity is always trying to pull us down. But what is life? Life is that inimitable unseen force, which constantly battles against this downward pull. The power of gravity does take over one fateful day. Till then, rejoice in every breath and maintain the harmonious flow of life by keeping the 'life cord' comfortably stretched within a healthy parameter.

Chapter 21

SLEEP RIGHT

Tension is who you think you should be.
Relaxation is who you are.
~ Chinese Proverb

The best position to sleep in is one that is comfortable and maintains the natural curvatures of the spine too. Sleep should relax the muscles and the nerves while ensuring that the discs stay free and decompressed. Muscles that may have tightened during the day should normalize. When all this happens, circulation improves and an environment for healing is created.

Many a time, the way we sleep becomes a cause for aches and pains during the day. Sometimes it also leads to fatigue and sleepiness. Despite that, we feel comfortable sleeping in that same posture only.

To cure the problems arising out of sleeping posture needs a change of habits. This is not an easy proposition, but doing this is the only way you can get rid of those problems. You can first adopt the changes at the time of going to bed. Slowly, start telling yourself this is how you need to sleep through the night. Our brain is smart enough to register positions that relieve or reduce pain. So, after a while, you will get into the habit of sleeping in a posture that is best-suited for your health. Remember that it helps to alternate between various ways of sleeping mentioned in this chapter. That way, the body does not get used to any one posture and is spared the trouble of bearing the pressure on the same points day after day.

Let us look at the various ways in which people are observed to sleep, what goes wrong and how we can adjust the position to take us towards the ideal way of lying down for our nightly rest.

Sleeping on the Belly

Only those with a flat back feel comfortable when they sleep on the belly. However, in the long run, they experience discomfort. Long hours of a curved pelvis lead to stiffness in the lower back. The discomfort doubles with a protruded belly. The lower back tends to sink in further.

People with weak abdominals should avoid sleeping on the belly because:

- The lower back sinks further in and downward. This causes extra pressure on the discs of the lower spine.

- It may cause swayback and neck sprain.

- It creates a twist in the cervical spine and the pelvis.

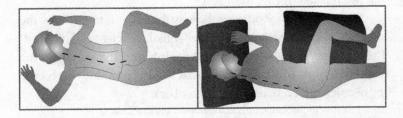

Sleeping on the belly (wrong); Supporting folded leg (right)

Solution

Use Support – People who suffer from chronic headaches or neck aches find relief when they correct this position and take the pressure off the neck and the pelvis. Those who find it difficult to change their 'tummy sleeping' posture can be safer by following these simple suggestions.

- Place a rolled towel or a small pillow under the abdomen to prevent a sag in the lower back.

- One knee can be bent towards the chest.

- The pillow below the head should be as flat as possible so that the neck does not get arched or twisted to one side.

At the same time, it is worth considering a change in the habit of belly sleeping. A conscious start can be to lie down on any side or on the back when you go to bed. Learn to relax in the newly acquired position. Give some time to the body to accept it and then gradually wean off from the old habit of belly sleeping.

Sleeping on the Back

Sleeping on the back significantly reduces the pressure on the back compared to sleeping on the stomach, as the weight is evenly distributed across the widest surface of the body. However, it is not uncommon to have complaints from people suffering from aches and pains even when they sleep in the supine position. The reason they feel stiff is because the muscles in the back are taut and not relaxed during the sleep.

Notice the pictures and see the way the pelvis is tilted. Since the lower back is overarched, the lower spinal muscles are tightened. The curvature puts pressure on the joints and the nerves of the back. This leads to a stiff and sore back in the morning, especially for people with an overarched lower back.

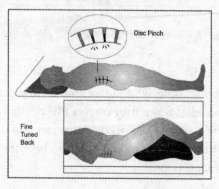

Sleeping on the back with tight muscles and sleeping stretched with a pillow under the knees

Solution

Sleep Stretched – We should sleep on the back in a neutral position where the muscles of the back are stretched comfortably and are not stiff or tight. This involves elongating the spine when we lie down. This resting position is comparable to a therapeutic traction.

- Lie down on your bed with your head resting on a pillow.

- Fold your knees with the feet flat on the bed.

- Hold your hips lightly with your palms, fingers facing down.

- Push the hips away from your lower back, towards your feet. This is the same as aligning the pelvis when we stand.

- Walk your shoulders down to take them away from the ears. Roll the shoulders down so they are rested on the bed.

- To stretch your neck, lift it off the pillow and stretch it away from the body. Maintain the extra length created as you gently place the head back on the pillow.

- Ease out. Straighten your legs. Keep the arms by the side, palms face the ceiling.

- Check your lower back again. It should not be arched up too high. You should be able to slide the fingers of one hand into the natural gap between the back and the bed. If the gap is too much, do all these steps with a pillow placed below your knees.

- If you have tight lower back muscles or suffer from backaches, place a medium-sized, firm pillow under the knees and the lower legs. Note that the pillow should not be too thick, too soft or too hard. This support stretches the back and reduces the arch. The padding also reduces the pressure on the spine and the discs.

Sleeping stretched has many advantages. Not only does it improve the quality of the sleep, it is also conducive to the spine.

It decompresses the discs and the spinal nerves, improves blood circulation and resets the resting length of the tight back muscles. The improvement in the breathing in this specific position is noteworthy.

Tips for Correct Pillow Usage
Make sure the head does not tip too far forward or too far behind. Both situations strain the neck. Place the pillow under the head in such a way that

- the neck is in a neutral position in line with the spine.

- the face is parallel to the ceiling.

- the forehead and the chin are at the same horizontal level.

Sleeping on Either Side

People who sleep on the side tend to lean forward from the top, so the top shoulder and the top hip fall ahead. This misaligns the said joints and twists the spine. If you are habituated to sleeping on one side, these guidelines will come in handy.

- Lie on any side with the hips and the knees bent.

- Elongate the waist by pushing the hips towards the feet to increase the distance between the hip and the armpit.

- If the lower back is rounded behind, lift the hips up slightly. Use your top hand to pull the fleshy part of the hip backward and reposition yourself down. Remember not to overarch the lower back.

- If the lower back is swayed or overarched, try to lengthen it while you retain a mild pelvic tilt.

- Place a firm pillow between your knees and legs to keep the hips, the pelvis and the spine aligned. The thickness of the pillow should be such that the top knee, leg and hip are exactly on top of the lower knee, leg and hip. This helps considerably, especially when in pain, as it takes off the pressure from the lower hip and also keeps the pelvis vertical. It maintains the curve of the spine and alleviates any pressure on the discs.

- Many people feel more comfortable with the lower leg straight. The upper knee is bent and placed on the bed with an unhealthy spinal twist. Place a pillow beneath the bent knee to prevent this undesirable twist.

- For those with a sag in the spine due to a narrow waist and wide hips, placing a small towel rolled under the waist helps support the spine.

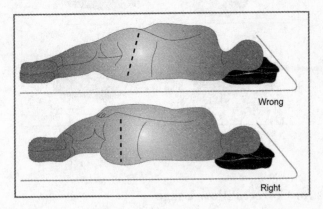

Wrong and right hip alignment

Solution
Stack the Joints Neatly –

- While sleeping on any side, the major joints of the body should stack on top of each other – knee on knee, hip on hip and foot on foot.

- When seen from the top, the head, the back, the hips and the feet should be in one line.

- The lower arm can be folded and placed comfortably on the bed or under the pillow.

- The top palm should rest on the top thigh.

- With the top shoulder rolled back, the nerves going from the neck to the arms do not get compressed. The upper shoulder should not get rounded or roll forward as this only reinforces the unhealthy habit of slumping.

- Alternate on each side to prevent muscular imbalance between the two sides of the body.

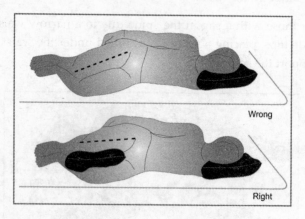

Stacking the joints with a pillow

Tips for Correct Pillow Usage

When we sleep on the side, there is a significant gap between the neck and the mattress due to the width of the shoulder. The head drops down creating a downward tilt in the spine at the neck. A correct pillow is of utmost importance to save the neck.

- The pillow should be firm and should provide proper support to the neck.

- It should be thick enough to span from the ears to the shoulders to keep the neck in line with the spine.

- The pillow should not be too thin. Otherwise, the head tilts down towards the mattress and the shoulders roll in, beating the purpose of taking a pillow in the first place.

- The pillow should not be too thick as the head would tilt up.

The pillow required thus depends on the anatomy, the length and the curvature of the neck. It also depends on the position in which a person prefers to sleep most of the time. The universal aim is to keep the neck in a neutral position – in line with the spine.

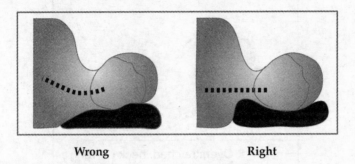

Wrong   **Right**

Head-neck alignment – Wrong and right ways

The Pillow Debate

It is commonly assumed that a pillow aggravates the pain of cervical spondylosis. This is a generalization as each person has different body proportions. Pillow selection may be compared to tailor made clothes. It is important to choose a pillow according to the alignment of the neck and the spine. The aim should be to keep the neck at a neutral position so that the muscles in the back of the neck are comfortable and do not get strained during the night. These muscles should get a gentle traction-like stretch with the help of a good pillow.

A good pillow should help neutralize the tightness and the altered curvature of the neck and the upper back. The pillow should certainly not perpetuate or increase the unhealthy curves. It should encourage the neck to stretch gently. A good pillow is firm enough to hold the baseline shape, yet soft enough to nurture a good sleep.

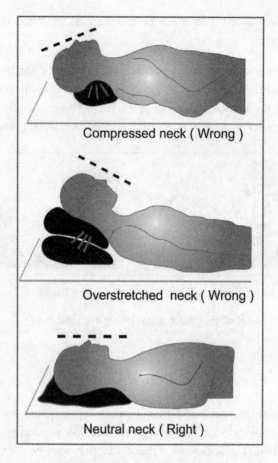

Compressed neck (Wrong)

Overstretched neck (Wrong)

Neutral neck (Right)

Wrong and right ways of using a pillow

Cervical rolls are made to support the natural curvature of the neck or to create one. Increased curvature is common due to the shortening of the back neck muscles. It is advisable to lengthen these muscles with additional support rather than curve the spine.

If the neck muscles are too tight and it is difficult to stretch them due to muscle spasms, cervical rolls can be used temporarily. It is better to support the neck rather than leave it unsupported. Yet, anything that exaggerates the cervical curvature should not be used. Over time, stretching the neck with the help of an appropriate pillow helps the most.

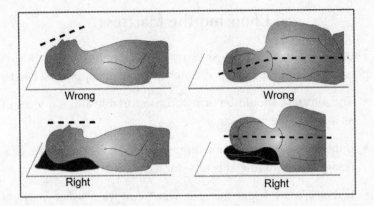

Sleeping without and with a pillow

The cervical roll should be such that it starts at the base of the skull and not at the top of the neck. A support that begins at the base of the skull will elongate the neck appropriately and avoid the cringe at the back of the neck. The thumb rule is that the forehead and the chin should be at the same level.

A quick recap of the ideal position of the pillow for different sleeping positions.

- Stomach sleepers need a very thin, flat pillow or no pillow at all. The pillow should not force an acute neck angle from behind.

- People who sleep on their backs need a softer pillow so that the head sinks in and is not pushed too far up.

- Side sleepers need firm, thicker pillows to fill the gap between the neck and the mattress.

- Even a rolled towel or bed sheet when placed in the curvature of the neck can give a balanced support. However, the head should not be allowed to fall back as this leads to overarching of the neck and causes more harm than good.

- While watching TV in bed or while reading, do not thrust the head forward. Instead, stack pillows one on top of each other to raise the body up from the waist.

Choosing the Mattress

The mattress we choose to sleep on plays an important role too. A person's specific body type dictates the type of support he needs.

- The mattress should be firm and comfortable and not too soft as it makes the body sag.

- If the mattress has become lumpy and the coils can be felt, or if it sags in the middle, it is time for a change.

- If the hips are wider than the waist, opt for a softer mattress to accommodate the width of the pelvis and allow the spine to remain neutral.

- If the hips and the waist are in a relatively straight line, a more rigid surface offers better support.

Getting Up from the Bed

No spring actions, please. The clock alarm wakes one up with a start and jerks the body out of bed. This can be hazardous and may precipitate problems. Remember springing out from the bed can cause injury to the spine and the discs.

All animals, even birds, stretch in the morning. It is our kind, the intellectuals, who are so driven by ambition and a fast-paced life that we forget the natural need of the body to stretch first thing in the morning. It is wise to ease out the tightness in the muscles that might have accrued due to sleeping in wrong postures.

First things first:

- Interlock your palms, turn them up and take them above your head.

- Give yourself a good, good-morning stretch by pointing your toes and interlocked hands away from the body. Breathe in comfortably and repeat.

- Turn to one side. Press the bed with the upper hand and push the trunk up as you sit.

- As you breathe in, stretch interlocked hands up towards the sky once again and get started for a great day!

Chapter 22

SAFE FORWARD BENDING

The mind's first step to self-awareness
must be through the body.
~ George A. Sheehan

It is worthwhile to observe farmers at work in the fields as they bend down on and off, clearing weeds, planting seeds and doing much more. Notice their backs as they toil. They bend for long hours without any problem because they maintain a forward bend by hinging at the hips and keep their backs flat through the bend. Strong muscles, that create a central groove over the spine along with well-placed shoulder blades, keep this laborious job from becoming a back-breaking affair.

The one action that can make or break even a strong back is a forward bend. Doctors will confirm that behind most cases of backaches, there is a history of lifting some heavy object incorrectly. Does that mean that we should never ever bend forward and lift an object? It is impractical and rather impossible to perform the daily chores without these common and essential actions; we have to bend and straighten many times a day. The question should not be: Should we bend or not?' It ought to be: How should we bend forward?'

Forward Bending: The Right Ways

When bending forward, you must keep the following points in mind:

Hinge at the Hip: A healthy forward bend involves a forward hinge at the hips with a straight lower back. The length of the back ought to be maintained all through the bend. Such a bend does not affect any disc anywhere in the spine. The discs remain decompressed and are not under any strain.

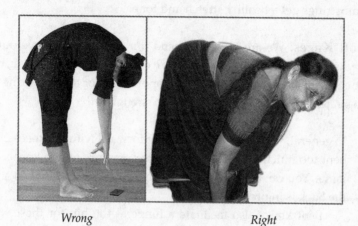

Wrong   *Right*

Bending forward – Wrong and right ways

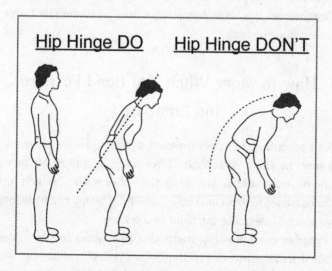

Hip hinge – Right and wrong ways

Wrong bending can be a threat to the back but a healthy bend at the hips is a beneficial exercise for the muscles of the back as they get a healthy stretch. Such a bend brings muscles that run along the length of the spine into action. This keeps the back aligned rather than rounded. As these muscles strengthen, the hamstrings get a healthy stretch and tone.

Soft Knees: We are taught to bend our knees to preserve our backs. This does preserve the back as it does not round. However, it stresses the knees and reduces the opportunity for the hamstrings to stretch and for the back muscles to strengthen.

In general, you must avoid bending forward with the knees bent too much as this can put undue pressure on the knee joints. You can bend knees for lifting heavy objects or when the back is injured or in pain.

Bent knees also facilitate a hinge at the hip for those with tight hamstrings. In such cases, tight hamstrings pull the sitting bones (to which they are attached) down. This forces the pelvis to tip backward. Bent knees ease the demand on the tight hamstrings and facilitate the hinge forward at the hips.

How to Move When You Bend Forward and Come Up?

In the beginning, a correct forward bend requires concentration and slow motion. With time, it becomes an automatic process. As the muscles stretch, we create flexibility with a hinged hip. It becomes easier to bend and stay in the bent position a little longer as we learn to decrease the bend in the knees.

Practise the following method a few times to get a feel of the ideal mechanism of bending forward and coming up. Teach yourself to apply it when you need to bend forward during the course of the day.

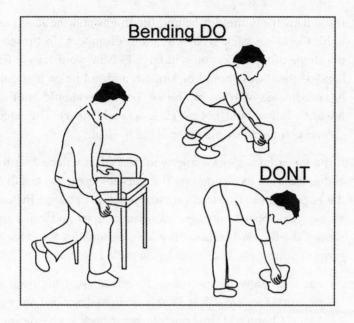

Bending forward – Right and wrong ways

- Stand with the feet parallel at hip-width distance. If the forward bend is deep, you can place your feet wider apart.

- Place the fingertips of one of your hands in the midline groove of your lower back. This is to monitor the bend.

- Place the edge (little finger side) of your other hand in the crease or the fold between the torso and the thigh. When you bend, feel the hinging on the hip joint on this hand.

- Unlock your knees and keep them soft. You can bend them as necessary to accommodate the tightness of your hamstrings.

- Start the bend from the hip joints. Feel your pelvis come forward as your back follows it.

- The fingertips of the hand on your lower back should not feel any change in the midline groove. If the groove begins to disappear or if it becomes deeper, straighten up a bit and proceed again.

- If the hamstring muscles behind the thighs and the knees are tight, the lower back groove tends to disappear. To preserve the shape of the back, you will have to bend your knees. The bend at the knees should be smooth and not jerky. It should be coordinated with the hip hinge. The knees should not turn inward (they should not go close to each other). The knees should point in the same direction as the feet.

- If the lower back groove begins to deepen, it reflects that the abdominals are weak and lax. The muscles along the length of the back begin to over-contract to deepen the groove. In such a case, remember to engage your inner corset and come up. Restart the forward bend with your core muscles activated to support your lower back from being pulled down.

  - For the safety of the neck, do not allow your neck to protrude forward. Glide your head in as described on page 136 in Chapter 14. Imagine that your neck is an extension of the spine and keep it aligned with the head, the neck and the shoulders in the same manner as you would when you stand.

- When you are ready to come up, engage your inner corset and start unhinging at the hip joints so that the trunk moves up along with the pelvis. The groove in the back should remain the same.

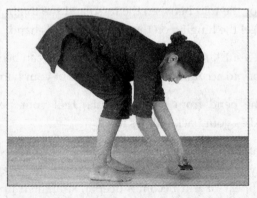

Safe forward bending

Backaches Related to Forward Bends

The above pointers are meant for unlearning old habits of bending and learning the correct method. If the lower back hurts when you bend forward, it means that the back muscles are in a state of spasm or contraction. Forward bends stretch the back muscles, making the back round or sway. This leads to pain. To keep the back supported and the lower spine discs safe, observe these safeguards:

- Navel in: Engage your inner corset before you begin to bend. This helps to maintain the torso as a single unit.

- Gentle bend at the knees: If the back still hurts, start with a small bend in the knees along with the inner core tone. Use bent knees till your back heals. Practise lower back stretches and abdominal strengthening exercises regularly. (For details, please refer to Chapter 12.)

- In case of an acute prolapsed disc, take rest to relax the back muscles and follow the doctor's advice. Apply these principles once the back has healed and you have been advised to resume normal activities.

Lifting Heavy Objects

Lifting heavy objects exerts further pressure on the joints of the spine. It is estimated that lifting a 12 kg weight with bent knees and a straight back puts around 140 kg of force on the bones of the spine. If the same weight is lifted with straight knees and bending from the waist, the force exerted on the back gets almost doubled. You can save your back all this anguish.

- Assess the load and its weight by pushing it with your foot. If it is too heavy, ask someone for help.

- Avoid bending and lifting anything first thing in the morning as one is more vulnerable to disc injury at that time.

- Go close to the load. The closer we are to the object, the lesser is the strain on the joints. The weight evenly distributes over the spine, the pelvis and the legs. Also, you are less likely to lose balance and fall. The pressure on the back increases when the distance from the object increases.

- Face the object. Do not venture to lift objects when the body is twisted. Most injuries caused while lifting objects occur when the spine is twisted. The remedy is to face the load before we lift the object. Lifting sideways is a definite 'NO'.

- Before the lift, tighten the abdominal muscles as much as you can. This accords a firm support to the lower back. So, take a deep breath and pull the navel in as much as you can, as if you are zipping up a pair of tight-fit trousers. Keep the abdominals drawn in when you lift or put the weight down. However, do not forget to breathe simultaneously!

- Do not bend from the waist. Bend the knees and the hips. This allows the larger muscles of the legs to work. If you bend from the waist to lift objects, the back muscles have to work twice as hard to do the job. In addition, if they are already compromised, the pressure gets transmitted to the discs – a dangerous proposition.

- Pick the load and bring it in close to the body. Push the ground firmly with both your feet as you straighten your legs.

- If you need to carry the load, keep the stomach muscles tight as you breathe.

- Maintain a neutral spine.

- As you carry the object, hold it as close to the body as possible. Again, the closer the object to the body, the lesser the strain on the spine and the muscles.

- Never raise a heavy object above the waist level.

- If you need to turn, do not twist at the waist with the object in your hands. Instead, turn your feet with small steps to turn the body.

- To lower the load, again bend your knees and hips. Stick the buttocks behind as you go down.

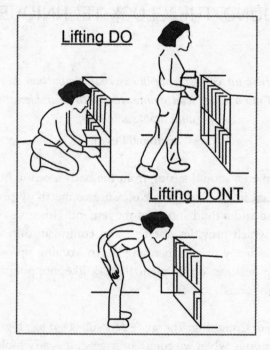

Lifting objects – Right and wrong ways

Shifting Furniture or Heavy Objects

The same body mechanics of a neutral spine hold good for pushing heavy objects. Keep the knees and the hips bent, as you face the object to be pushed.

Chapter 23

ROUND-THE-CLOCK TECHNIQUES

Right discipline consists, not in external compulsion, but in the habits of mind which lead spontaneously to desirable rather than undesirable activities.

~ Bertrand Russell

Movements should spring from the body's centre of gravity, placed just below the navel. Core connectivity provides a stable base and a fluid source of movement. This gives a central support, which provides strength and control in difficult tasks like lifting heavy objects, bending down, coming up erect from a bending position, doing manual work like mopping the floor, digging on farms, etc.

Sneezing or Coughing: The spine gets subjected to a high level of pressure torque when we cough or sneeze. It is advisable to lean back slightly or stay erect during bouts of sneezing and coughing. Bending forward during these bouts can trigger or worsen an injury.

Shopping: Avoid carrying a heavy shopping bag in one arm. Divide the contents in two or more bags and distribute the weight evenly between the bags. Carry the bags in both arms. Use a shopping cart, wherever available.

- Bend your elbows and use the strength of your upper arms to carry the weight. This protects the wrists and the shoulders from bearing the brunt.

- Keep your upper back wide to create more stability.

- Avoid leaning on one side.

- Keep the bags close to your body.

Cleaning and Vacuuming: When you use a vacuum cleaner to clean the floor, turn your feet in the direction you want to clean rather than twisting the waist. Also, keep the arms as close to the body as possible instead of reaching out. Use the full length of the rod of the vacuum cleaner or the broom to facilitate cleaning.

Making the Bed: When you change bed spreads, do not bend at the waist. Instead, bend at the hips. Keep the knees bent as you go about the work. Do not lean over too far. Sit or stand on the side you are working on. It is also convenient to kneel on one or both the knees while making the bed.

Cycling: Cycling can be injurious if done with a rounded back. If done with proper body alignment, it is unlikely to cause injury. Cycling helps strengthen the hip flexors or the front muscles of the thighs. However, without complementary stretches, these muscles shorten. This gives a pull on the pelvis and the lumbar spine, overarching the lower back.

- Make sure you do some warm up exercises, especially for your legs before cycling.

- Select a bike which is adjustable as per the body structure. Trail bikes allow better posture than racing bikes.

- The seat should be such that when the pedal is the farthest away, the legs straighten without locking/hyperextending the knees.

- The handle should be adjusted so that you do not have to lean on it while cycling. While leaning, not only does the back slump, but the head also pushes forward, which strains the neck and the back.

- Make sure you do some leg stretches after you are done cycling. Include stretches for the front, back, inner and outer sides of the thighs.

Exercising: Any sport is an enjoyable activity for those interested. However, awareness of balance between using a muscle and stretching it during the activity is very important.

- **Weight Training Programs**: These should be adopted with caution or under the supervision of an experienced trainer for a balanced workout. Otherwise, weights may strengthen the existing misalignments!

   Engaging the deep postural muscles while holding weights is important, as many sculpted bodies have weak backs and disc prolapses.

- **Dance Classes**: It is good to let your hair down and dance your heart out as long as the muscles are correctly engaged. Often, to get the dance step right, muscles get punished with wrong movement.

- **Walking on Machines**: To train our cardiovascular system, we challenge ourselves by an increase in the speed and slope of the walking space. We also bang our heels in the process, which aggravates the impact and misaligns the knees. Nothing can replace natural walking in the open with proper footwear. It is a panacea for the mind and the body.

- **Deceptive Looks**: Six or eight-pack abs and over-sized biceps are commonly equated with fitness. Over-strengthened abs may make the abdominal wall so tight that there is a risk of distorting the body alignment. Not to mention the ill-effects on breathing. The muscle groups on the back, the sides and the front of the body balance the effects of the abdominals and need attention too.

Post-Partum (After Delivery) Care: Pregnancy related posture is a topic vast enough to deserve an entire book. Needless to say, the following tips are not exhaustive. These are just quick tips to avoid common back pain after child birth, as the over-stretched abdominal muscles go weak. The sagging abdomen cannot support the back and therefore creates a forward pull on the back. The arch of the back thus exaggerates and puts pressure on the joints, the muscles and the nerves. Lifting and carrying the baby adds pressure on the back.

- **Lifting Your Baby:** Bend your knees and hips and tighten the abdominals before you lift your baby. Avoid a twist in your torso when you have lifted the baby.

- **Carrying Your Baby:** The general tendency is to lean back when you hold the baby to compensate for the baby's weight. This puts pressure on the back and results in lower back pain. So, when you carry your baby, pull your abdomen in slightly, tuck the tail-bone down and keep the back straight. Also, switch sides from time to time.

- **Breast Feeding:** Do not slouch or round the upper back when you feed your baby. Instead, sit erect and bring the baby closer to the body. Place a pillow on your lap and rest the baby on a pillow instead of holding your little one in the arms.

Chapter 24

FAQs

Judge a man by his questions rather than by his answers.

~ Voltaire

i. **There is nothing I can do about my pain. I am aging and this pain is a part of the process.**

Aging is unavoidable as every birthday marks another year gone by. Come early forties and a gradual loss of muscle mass sets in. We lose this mass by about 2-3 kilograms every 10 years, making the bones vulnerable. The young generation too is aging pre-maturely as the sedentary lifestyle encourages functional aging.

This does not mean we have to spend our sunset years in pain. Our health is in our control to a large extent. We can slow down the process of aging of our muscles by taking good care of them.

ii. **I have been advised to stand with straight legs. Why should I micro bend my knees when standing?**

Those with hyper-extended knees tend to have weaker muscles, causing the legs to give in. As a result more body weight is borne directly by the knee joints. This puts extra pressure behind the knees, shifts the weight of the body on the heels and causes the pelvis to tip forward. Thus, it is important to bend the knees gently.

Standing with the feet parallel helps solve this problem. It holds the knees in good stead. It also repositions the weight towards the ball of the foot and tilts the pelvis to a vertical position.

iii. **I cannot breathe while the navel is pulled in.**

The muscles in the back and the abdomen should be comfortably held, and not be taut and tense. If the navel is pulled too far back and in, breathing gets hampered. The navel pull aims to bring back the baseline tone in the muscles, which should enhance and improve breathing. A core tone and awareness brings about a smooth, quiet, relaxed and flowing breathing.

iv. **When I pull my shoulders back, I feel pain.**

You might feel a pinch in the shoulder blades when you try to open the chest. This happens when the action of taking the shoulders behind is overpowering. Such a motion actually immobilizes the chest and the back and can restrict breathing too. Pinched shoulder blades constrict freedom of movement in the arms and the upper body.

Widen your shoulders on the sides laterally, instead of pushing them behind too much. This gives the chest room to expand well. Also, make sure that you maximize the distance between your shoulders and your ears.

v. **When I do the Head Glide, I cannot breathe.**

It is very likely that you tuck your chin in towards the chest when you glide your head. When the chin is tucked in too deep such that it touches the chest, it presses upon the airways and hampers breathing. Overdoing any action is incorrect; maintaining a fine balance is valuable. Imagine there is a thread pulling you up from the topmost part of the head. This thread pulls through the back of the head and through the spine. Now, the chin neither points up nor squeezes in too hard. The correct position should be relaxed, not forced.

vi. Does bracing help?

Bracing any joint or body part restricts its movements. Initially it could prove helpful to reduce the pain as the tight muscles relax. But in the long run, bracing does more harm by making the muscles and the joints less resilient. Dysfunction gets multiplied. Active muscle tone is the best natural brace to protect the bones and the joints.

vii. I should not bend forward as I have backache. Is that right?

Forward bends should be avoided only in the acute phase of a herniated disc and other pathological conditions. As the back heals, the muscle spasms resolve and pain decreases to a comfortable level. At this stage, it is beneficial to do some gradual and calculated forward bends the correct way. If the muscles that allow forward bends are not allowed to perform their natural obligations, they stiffen to further exacerbate the painful condition.

Chapter 25

INSTANT RELIEF MANTRAS
24 x 7 Posture Awareness

Self-knowledge is the great power by which we comprehend and control our lives.
~ Vernon Howard

You have a good posture if there is an inherent sense of ease, natural grace and a lack of effort in any position. The guidelines below have been meticulously drawn for better comprehension.

Toes In, Heels Out: The feet when placed on the ground should be parallel, along their outer edges. The arches of the feet should be well formed and pronounced.

Knees Unlocked: Knees should not be pushed far behind but should be soft and centred. Do not bend them too much either.

Hip Clench: Gently squeeze your hip muscles. You should feel tall and energetic. Do not overdo to pinch the lower back.

Navel In: Pull the navel in by just half an inch to one inch. This should enhance your breaths and make your lower back feel supported. This along with the Hip Clench will automatically tuck your tail-bone down.

Head Glide: Slide your head behind so that the chin is parallel to the floor. Do not take your chin towards the chest such that it restricts your breathing. The back of your neck should feel elongated and relaxed.

The muscles of the body should have a baseline tone. The calf muscles, the front thigh muscles or the quadriceps and the buttock muscles should be used correctly in all activities, more so in the most common activities like walking and sitting.

The above guidelines have been logically enumerated for best effect. Imbibing these rudiments will motivate you to achieve a healthy and graceful body posture. This will reflect in the mirror and translate into compliments. This ego boost is the best incentive you can earn to continue on this journey. You may disconnect many times, but as soon as you reconnect, you will realize the benefits. Try, try till you succeed. I am positive that every sincere effort will be graciously awarded.

ABOUT THE AUTHOR

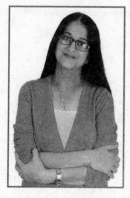

Dr Renu Mahtani, MD, is the founder of Param Yoga (www.paramyoga.in). She is a practicing physician and an adroit yoga therapist who has been associated with the Intensive Cardiac Care Unit of a leading hospital in Pune. Her journey eventually led her to research alternative healing practices, including avant-garde, potent and globally acclaimed yoga techniques.

Today, her medical practice is based on a holistic approach that combines minimal, necessary medications with lifestyle guidance on posture alignments and natural diet. She combines these with nutritional therapy and breath therapy along with mind management tips, with far-reaching benefits.

The author's workshops, along with her heartfelt oration, have brought wellness to several corporate organizations. Her workshops address various issues, from posture and office yoga to Pranayama for stress relief to managing chronic lifestyle ailments.

Dr Mahtani is the author of *The Ultimate Indian Diet Book*. Her last book Power Pranayama, which deals with the healing potential of breath, is a much-acclaimed work and has been translated in four languages.

With a vision of "the best possible health for all" and perpetual warmth in her heart, Dr Renu Mahtani lives by Robert Frost's lines, "I have promises to keep, and miles to go before I sleep."